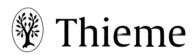

Practical Breast Pathology

Tibor Tot, M.D.
Department of Pathology and Clinical Cytology
Falun Central Hospital
Falun, Sweden

László Tabár, M.D.
Professor
Department of Mammography
Falun Central Hospital
Falun, Sweden

Peter B. Dean, M.D.
Professor
Department of Diagnostic Radiology
University Central Hospital
Turku, Finland

407 illustrations

Thieme
Stuttgart · New York

Library of Congress Cataloging-in-Publication Data is available from the publisher.

Important Note: Medicine is an ever-changing science undergoing continual development. Research and clinical experience are continually expanding our knowledge, in particular our knowledge of proper treatment and drug therapy. Insofar as this book mentions any dosage or application, readers may rest assured that the authors, editors, and publishers have made every effort to ensure that such references are in accordance with *the state of knowledge at the time of production of the book.*

Nevertheless this does not involve, imply, or express any guarantee or responsibility on the part of the publishers in respect of any dosage instructions and forms of application stated in the book. *Every user is requested to examine carefully* the manufacturer's leaflets accompanying each drug and to check, if necessary in consultation with a physician or specialist, whether the dosage schedules mentioned therein or the contraindications stated by the manufacturers differ from the statements made in the present book. Such examination is particularly important with drugs that are either rarely used or have been newly released on the market. Every dosage schedule or every form of application used is entirely at the user's own risk and responsibility. The authors and publishers request every user to report to the publishers any discrepancies or inaccuracies noticed.

© 2002 Georg Thieme Verlag,
Rüdigerstraße 14, D-70469 Stuttgart, Germany
Thieme New York, 333 Seventh Avenue,
New York, N.Y. 10001 USA

Typesetting by primustype Robert Hurler GmbH
D-73274 Notzingen, Germany

Printed in Germany by Grammlich, Pliezhausen

ISBN 3-13-129431-0 (GTV)
ISBN 0-86577-091-6 (TNY)   1 2 3 4 5

This book is dedicated to Mária, Viktória, and Kirsti

Preface

Radiologists, surgeons, oncologists, and other specialists working with diseases of the breast can perform far more effectively when they have a firm understanding of breast pathology. Fortunately, it is only the pathologist who needs to make histologic diagnoses. This book strives to provide the information which the non-pathologist needs to know and the pathologist should provide about breast diseases, without burdening the reader with details relevant only to the pathologist. Our approach emphasizes mammographic–pathologic correlation, explaining why two radiologists have joined a pathologist to write this book.

The material presented in this book has come exclusively from the Departments of Pathology and Mammography of the Central Hospital of Falun, Sweden, with patient follow-up exceeding 25 years. A collection of more than 3000 breast cancer cases with mammographic, specimen radiology, and large-section pathology correlation has been the source of our material, which includes several hundred cases with additional thick-section pathology.

Interdisciplinary diagnosis and treatment of breast diseases is slowly but irrevocably becoming accepted as the new golden standard for patient care. It requires an additional investment in time and effort, which is soon repaid by smoother delivery of care and far fewer iatrogenic complications. Interdisciplinary breast teamwork is a dynamic and demanding process, the ultimate reward of which is a significant improvement in patient care. This book has been written to assist in the implementation of interdisciplinary breast teamwork, to help the radiologist and pathologist communicate with each other, and to provide a framework for everyday cooperation within the breast team.

The Authors

Contents

Chapter 1

Normal Breast Tissue
or Fibrocystic Change?

The mammary gland, like all glandular organs, consists of parenchyma and stroma. The parenchyma contains ducts (Fig. 1.**1**) and lobules (Fig. 1.**2**), which are separated from the stroma by a continuous basement membrane (Fig. 1.**3**). The entire parenchyma (with the exception of the terminal parts of the lactiferous ducts) consists of a single inner layer of epithelial cells and an outer layer of myo-epithelium (Fig. 1.**4**). Only the epithelial cells contain estrogen and progesterone receptors in their nuclei (Fig. 1.**5**).

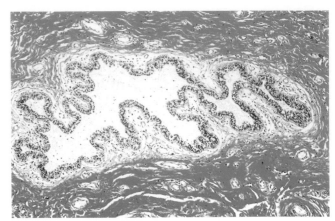

Fig. 1.**1**

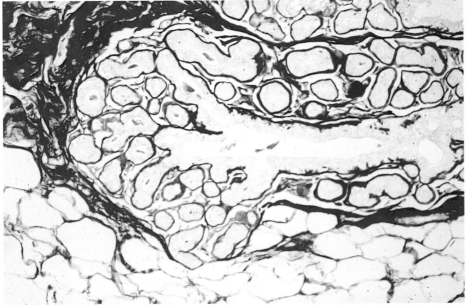

Fig. 1.**2**

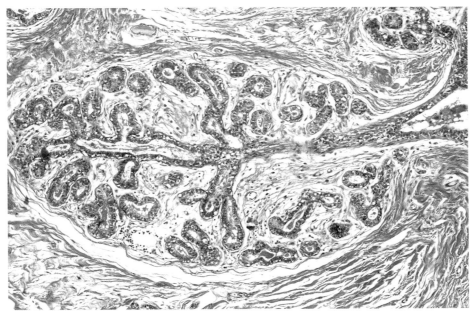

Fig. 1.**3**

The stroma consists of fibrous tissue and adipose tissue containing lymph vessels, blood vessels, and nerves. More specialized within the lobules and surrounding the ducts, the stroma can be divided into intralobular (mucin-rich, "active") and interlobular stroma (see Fig. 1.**16**).

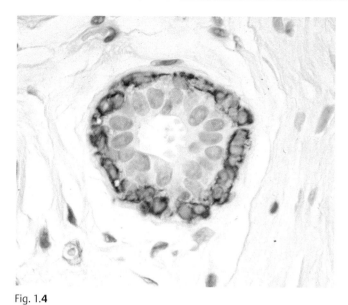

Fig. 1.4

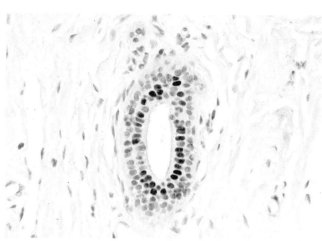

Fig. 1.5

The nipple is the origin of 15 to 25 lactiferous ducts, which branch into segmental, subsegmental, and terminal ducts that with the associated lobules comprise 15 to 25 lobes. The terminal duct and the associated lobule are collectively referred to as the Terminal Ductal-Lobular Unit (TDLU), which is the most important functional unit and the place of origin of most pathologic processes in the breast (Figs. 1.6 and 1.7).

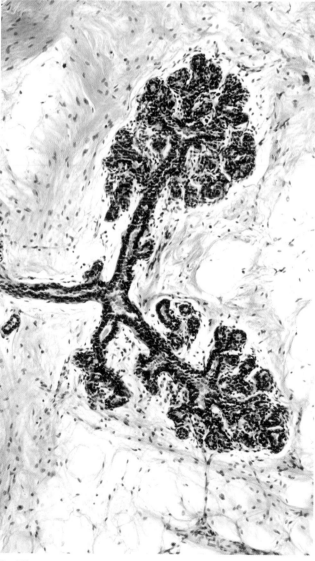

Fig. 1.6

Fig. 1.7

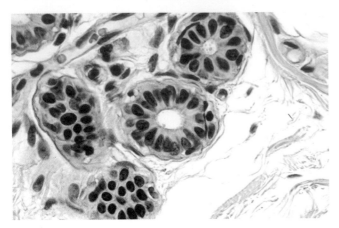

Fig. 1.8

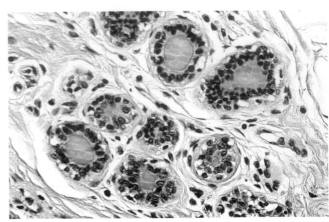

Fig. 1.9

At the beginning of the menstrual cycle, the lobules are relatively small and contain only a minimal amount of secretion, if any, in the lumina of the acini (Figs. 1.8 and 1.11). During the secretory phase of the cycle, the acini produce eosinophilic secretions and the intralobular stroma becomes edematous (Fig. 1.9). Around the time of menstruation, the myoepithelium becomes vacuolated and undergoes apoptosis (Fig. 1.10).

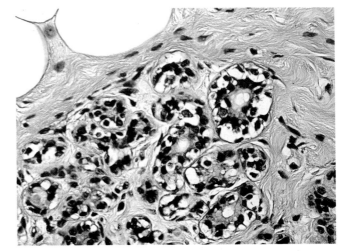

Fig. 1.10

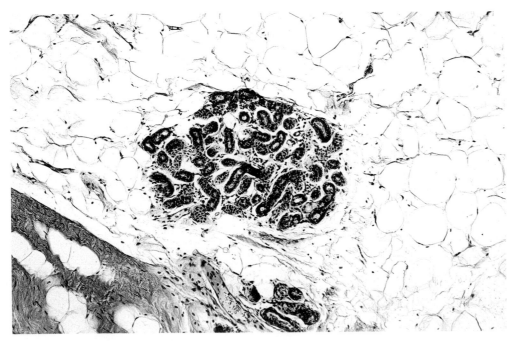

Fig. 1.11

Normal breast – number of acini/lobule

Acini / lobule

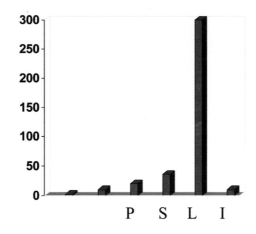

* personal observations

Fig. 1.**12**

P – proliferative phase of the menstrual cycle
S – secretory phase of the menstrual cycle
L – lactation
I – involution

The most obvious changes are seen during the last trimester of pregnancy and during lactation when the TDLUs are enlarged, the number of acini per lobule increases greatly (Fig. 1.**12**), the cytoplasm in the epithelial cells becomes vacuolated, and rich secretions are produced in large quantities (Fig. 1.**13**).

Fig. 1.**13**

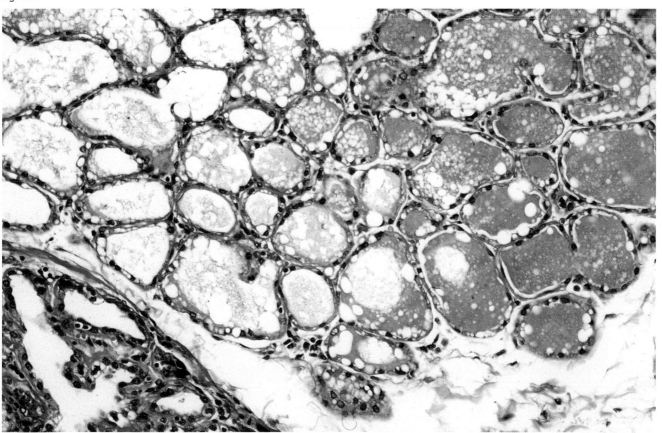

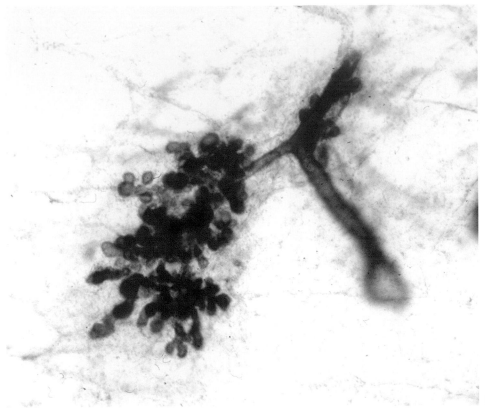

Fig. 1.**14**

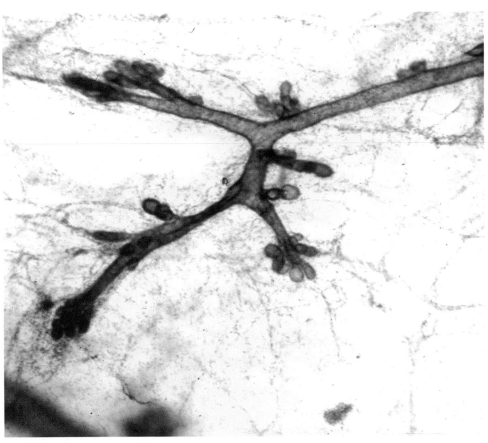

Fig. 1.**15**

Around the time of menopause, but often earlier, involution of the breast tissue occurs.
Involution of the parenchyma results in a diminished
number of acini/lobules, lobules, and ducts (compare
Fig. 1.**14** showing a functioning lobule with Fig. 1.**15** showing an involuted lobule, thick-section images).

Figure 1.**16** shows a TDLU with normal mucin-rich intralobular stroma. Involution of the intralobular stroma is accompanied either by infiltration of fatty tissue (Fig. 1.**17**) or by fibrosis (Fig. 1.**18**). The same is true for the interlobular stroma.

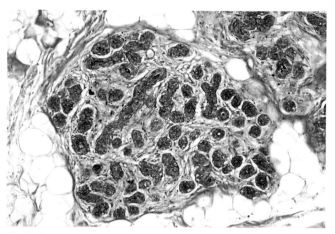

Fig. 1.**16**

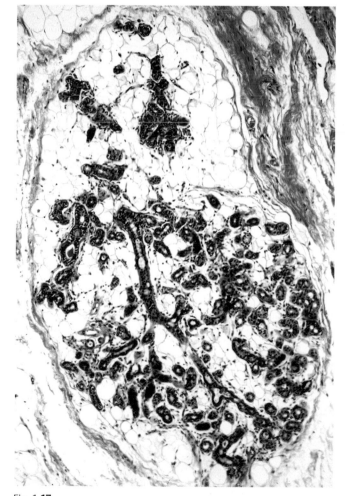

Fig. 1.**17**

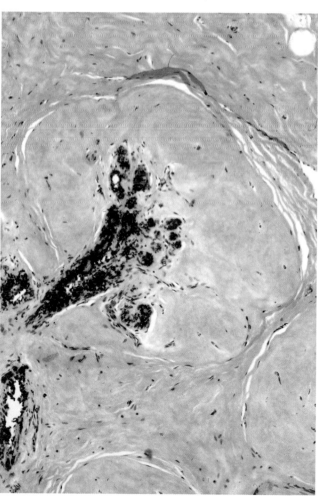

Fig. 1.**18**

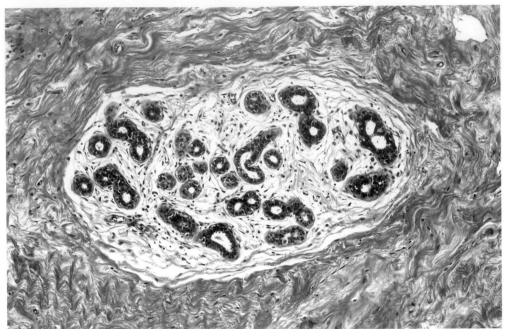

Fig. 1.**19**

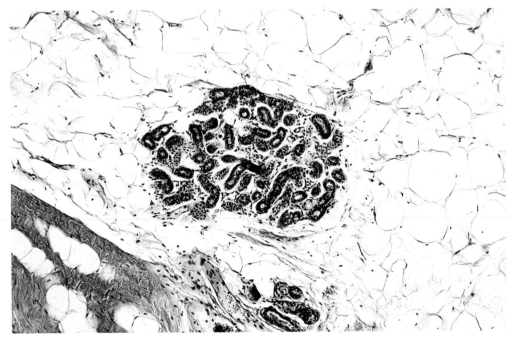

Fig. 1.**20**

The involution of the parenchyma and the interlobular and intralobular stroma is not necessarily a synchronized process. Functioning lobules can be seen in the presence of interlobular stroma that has undergone fibrous involution (Fig. 1.**19**) or has been replaced by fat (Fig. 1.**20**).

The intralobular and the interlobular stroma may undergo either fibrous or fatty involution in varying combinations (Figs. 1.**21**, 1.**22**, and 1.**23**).

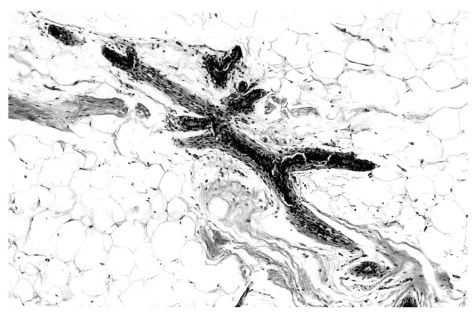

Fig. 1.**21**

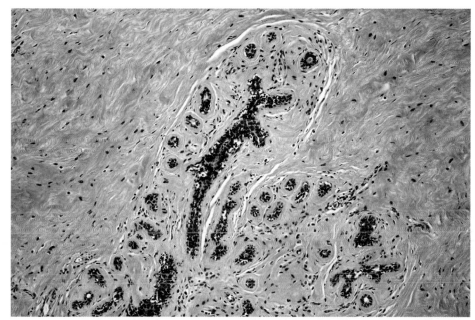

Fig. 1.**22**

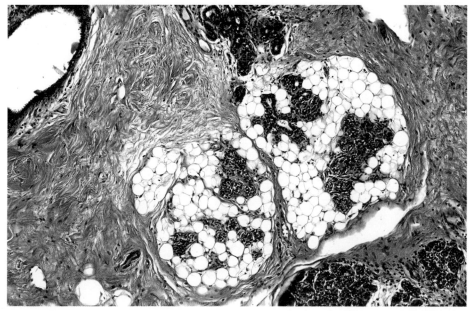

Fig. 1.**23**

The lobules may exhibit a deviated morphology as compared with that described previously. This phenomenon is called Aberration of Normal Development and Involution (ANDI). Some examples of ANDI:

– Apocrine metaplasia (Fig. 1.**25**) with large cells having granulated eosinophilic cytoplasm (as compared with normal epithelium, Fig. 1.**24**)
– Clear-cell change (Fig. 1.**26**)
– Eosinophilic change (Fig. 1.**27**), appearance of cells with eosinophilic cytoplasm among the cells of the usual type

– Lactational change (Fig. 1.**28**), milk-producing lobules in the breast of nonpregnant, nonlactating women
– Fibroadenomatoid change (Fig. 1.**29**) with proliferation of the intralobular stroma and distortion of the acini
– Microcystic involution (Fig. 1.**30**, galactography image; Fig. 1.**31**, thick-section image; and Fig. 1.**32**) if involution of the lobules (diminished number of acini) is associated with dilatation of the acini

A common type of ANDI is adenosis, which is described in detail in Chapter 6.

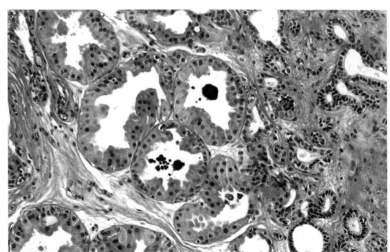

Fig. 1.**25**

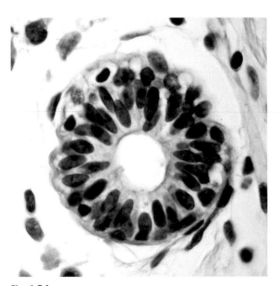

Fig. 1.**24**

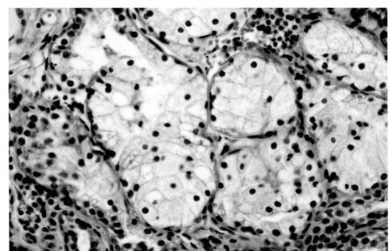

Fig. 1.**26**

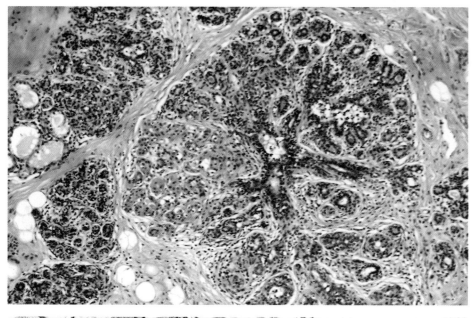

Fig. 1.**27**

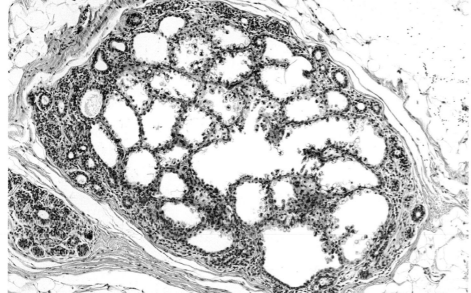

Fig. 1.**28**

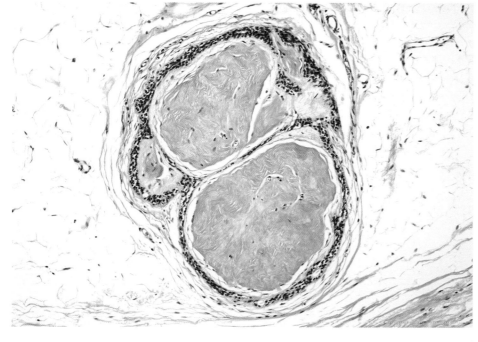

Fig. 1.**29**

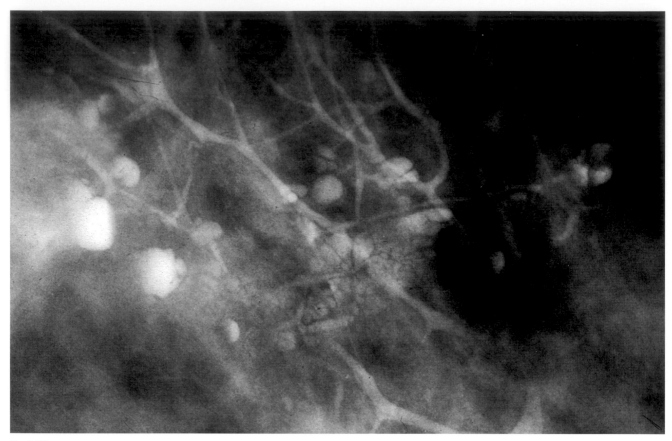

Fig. 1.**30**

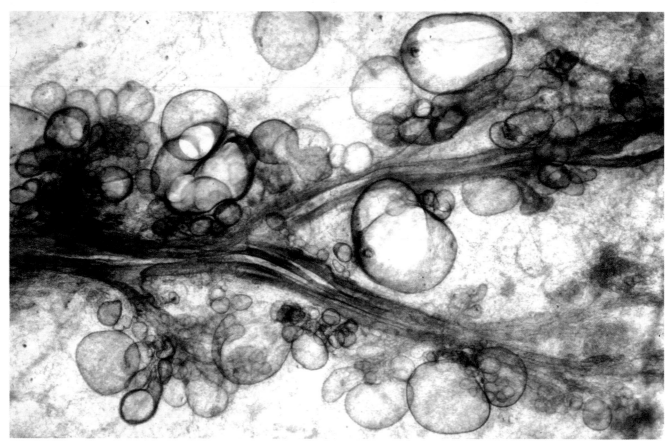

Fig. 1.**31**

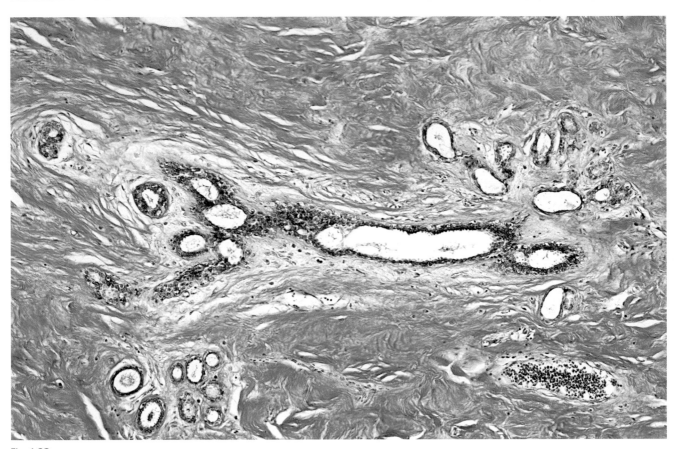

Fig. 1.**32**

Some ANDIs represent changes predominantly of the phenotype of the epithelial cells and may lead to accumulation of secretion in the lobule, which in turn may calcify. Other forms of ANDIs represent architectural changes within the lobules, leading to marked enlargement of the TDLUs. The calcifications or the enlarged TDLUs may be mammographically or clinically detected, causing anxiety for the patient and differential diagnostic problems for the radiologist.

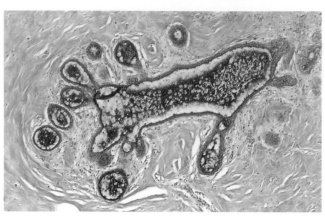

Fig. 1.**33**

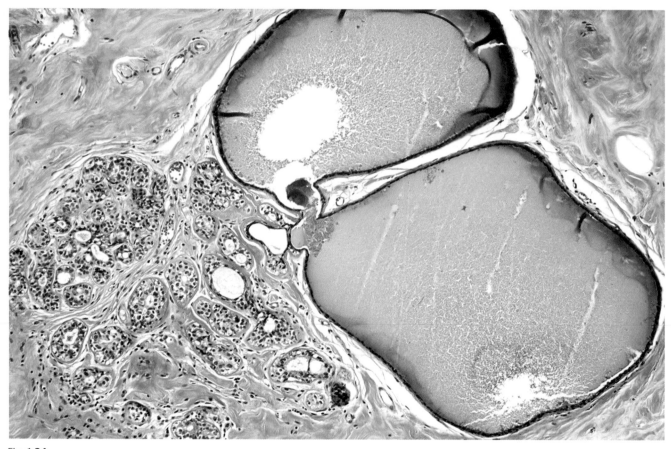

Fig. 1.**34**

The histologically "normal" breast tissue may show numerous aberrations, many of which cannot be detected by clinical or radiologic examination. If these lesions are sufficiently large to be radiologically or clinically detected and, especially when symptomatic, they are more appropriately called "fibrocystic change," which is still a variation of normal breast morphology.

The difference between ANDIs and fibrocystic change is more quantitative than qualitative. It is impossible to draw a sharp line between microcystic involution and cysts (Figs. 1.**33** and 1.**34**) or between fibroadenomatoid change and fibroadenoma (Figs. 1.**35** and 1.**36**).

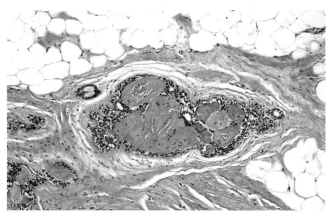

Fig. 1.**35**

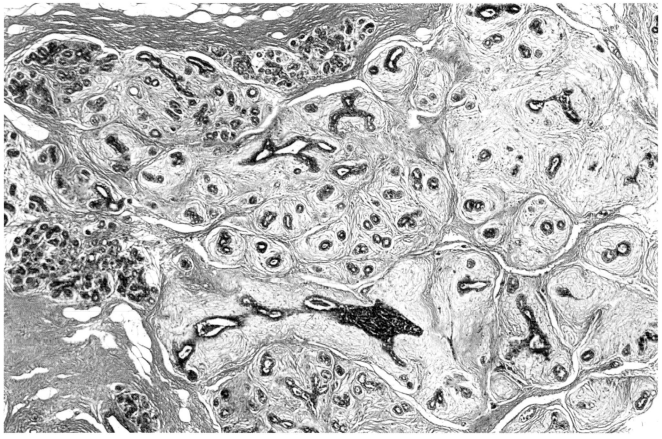

Fig. 1.**36**

The distinction between "normal" or "pathologic" depends on the method of examination. Histology is an extremely sensitive method and may detect many clinically and prognostically unimportant details, which are best characterized as variations and aberrations of the normal breast morphology.

The normal breast tissue contains lobules typical of both the proliferative and secretory and menstrual phases of the menstrual cycle, different combinations of involutional changes, and different ANDIs all at the same time. Consequently, normal breast tissue offers the interested examiner a variable and fascinating picture under the microscope (Figs. 1.**37**–1.**41**; Fig. 1.**40**, thick-section image).

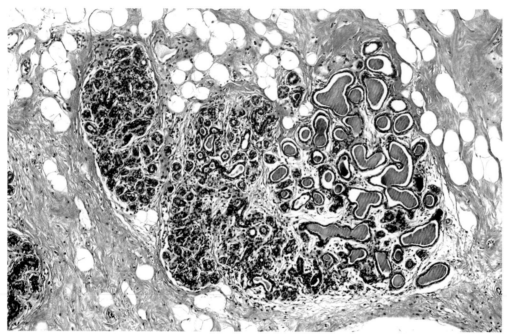

Fig. 1.**37**

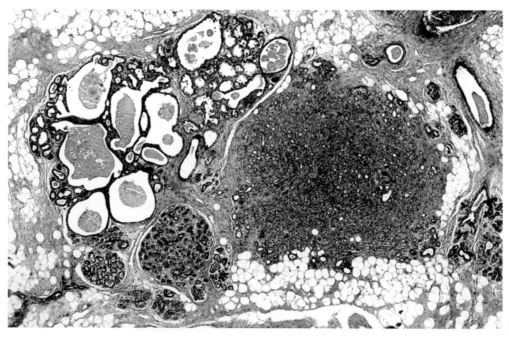

Fig. 1.**38**

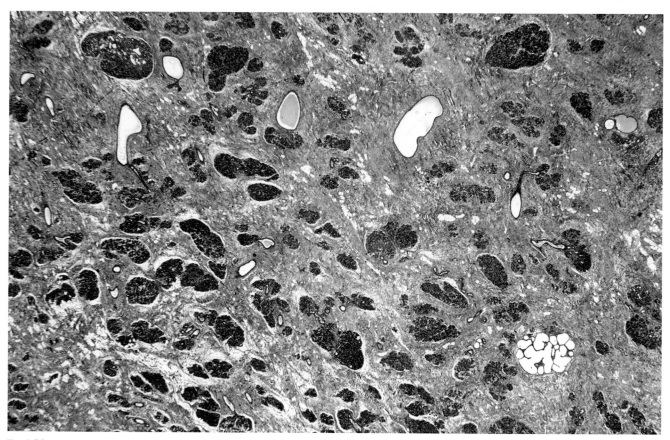

Fig. 1.**39**

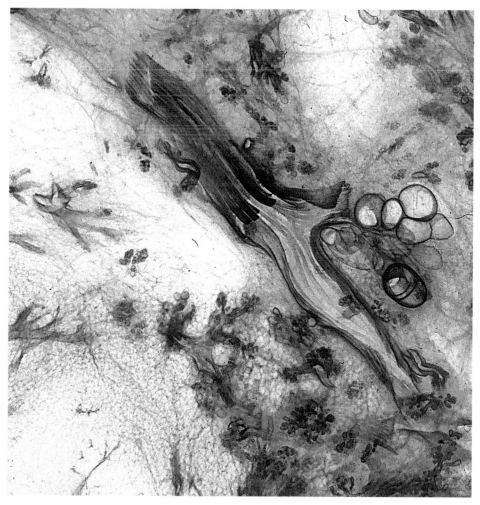

Fig. 1.**40**

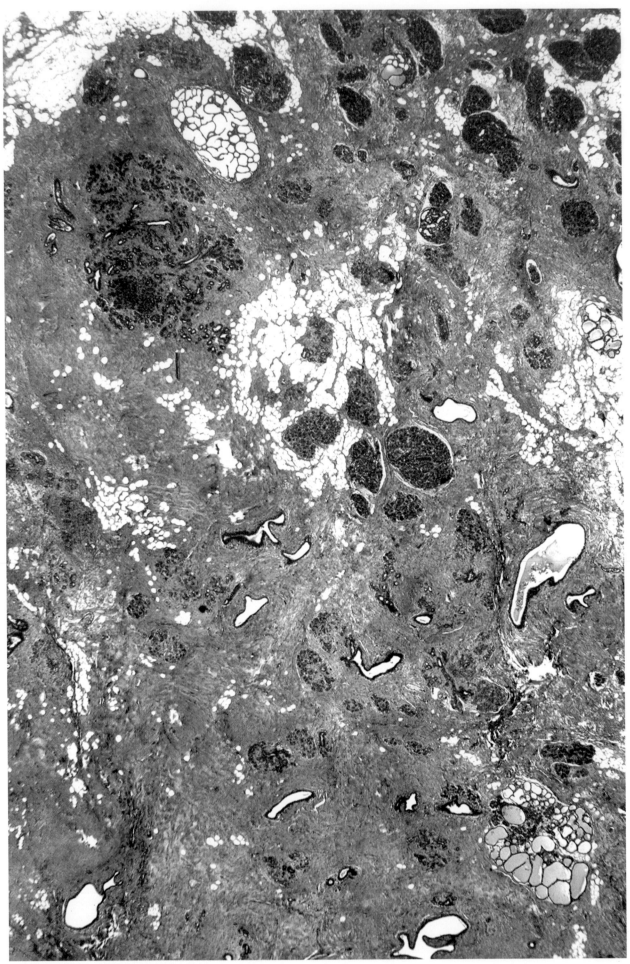

Fig. 1.**41**

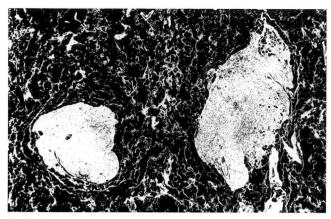

Fig. 1.**42**

The mammogram represents a black-and-white summation of the morphologic details of the breast. The lobules are visible on a high-quality mammogram as 1-to-2-mm nodular densities. Only the silhouettes of the lobules are seen, not the histologic details. A radiologic nodular density may represent a spectrum of histologic changes within the TDLU (Figs. 1.**42**–1.**44**). The radiologic linear densities correspond to ducts, fibrous strands, and vessels (Fig. 1.**45**).

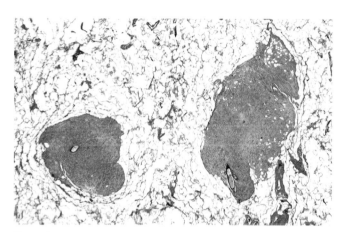

Fig. 1.**43**

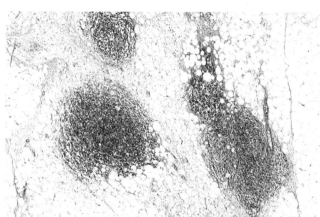

Fig. 1.**44**

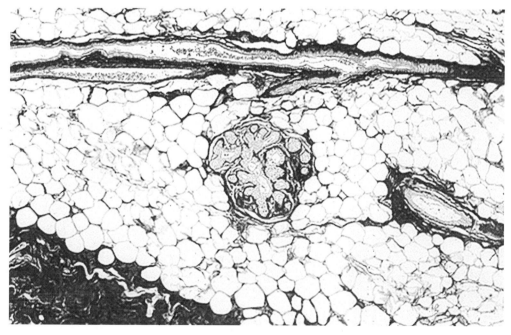

Fig. 1.**45**

Despite the variability of the histologic picture, the mammographic patterns of the normal breast can be properly classified in only five categories as described by Tabár, Gram and Tot. The basic factor determining the mammographic pattern of the normal breast is the interrelation between the radiopaque fibrous tissue and the radiolucent fatty tissue in the interlobular stroma.

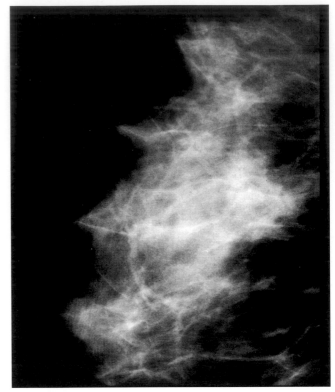

Mammographic pattern I is characterized by Cooper ligaments as well as a harmonic distribution of fatty and fibrous tissue (Figs. 1.46–1.48).

Fig. 1.46

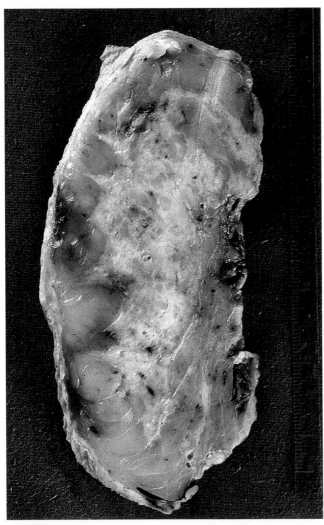

Fig. 1.47

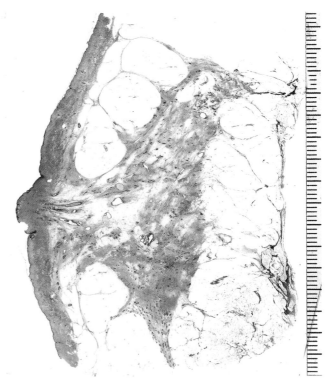

Fig. 1.48

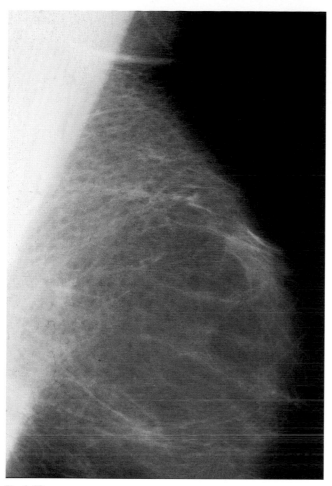

Fig. 1.**49**

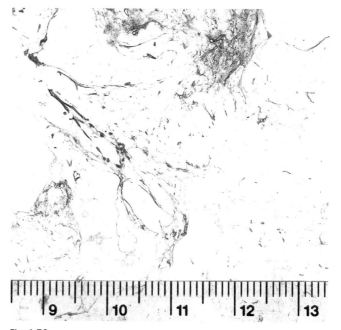

Fig. 1.**50**

Mammographic pattern II represents breast tissue replaced by fatty tissue with only a few remaining TDLUs (Figs. 1.**49** and 1.**50**).

Pattern I develops over time into pattern II through fatty involution. Hormone replacement therapy may convert pattern II back to pattern I. The mammographic pattern of the normal breast is often characterized as intermediate between patterns I and II or as "involuting pattern I."

Pattern III is characterized by a relatively fibrotic area behind the nipple when the remainder of the breast has been replaced by adipose tissue (Fig. 1.**51**). The same pattern can be produced by advanced ductectasia.

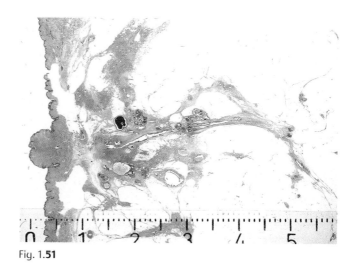

Fig. 1.**51**

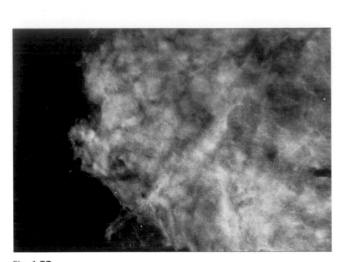

Fig. 1.**52**

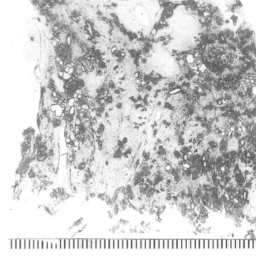

Fig. 1.**53**

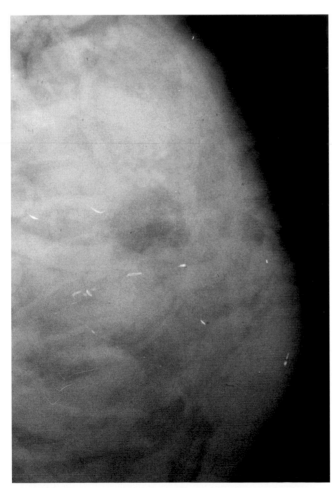

Fig. 1.**54**

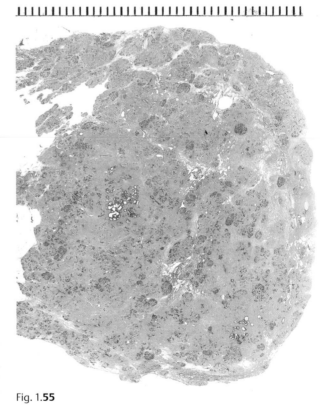

Fig. 1.**55**

Pattern IV is dominated by somewhat enlarged nodular densities, approximately 3 to 5 mm in size (Figs. 1.52 and 1.53). These densities usually represent different ANDIs, but focal involution of the interlobular stroma with small islands of remaining fibrous tissue may present the same picture (see Fig. 1.43).

Pattern V shows a radiopaque density over the entire gland corresponding to a more collagenous interlobular stroma (Figs. 1.54 and 1.55). Radiologic details (nodular or linear densities) are poorly seen; active and/or atrophic parenchyma may be hidden within this density.
Patterns IV and V are stable and do not change during the woman's lifetime.

Conclusions

Comprehensive knowledge of the variations of normal breast morphology enables the pathologist to avoid over-diagnosing normal variations as pathologic processes.

Clinical and radiologic diagnoses assist the pathologist in the delineation of normal tissue from fibrocystic change.

The particular mammographic pattern of breast tissue is an important aid for the pathologist. Detection of pathologic changes in breasts with patterns I, II, and III is relatively easy, but a more detailed histologic analysis of macroscopically and radiologically normal breast tissue is necessary in patients with patterns IV and V.

References

1 Vogel PM, et al. The correlation of histological changes in the human breast with the menstrual cycle. *Am J Pathol.* 1981;104:23–34.
2 Longacre TA, Bartow SA. A correlative morphologic study of human breast and endometrium in menstrual cycle. *Am J Surg Pathol.* 1986;10(6):382–393.
3 Hughes LE, et al. Aberrations of normal development and involution (ANDI): a new perspective on pathogenesis and nomenclature of benign breast disorders. *Lancet.* 1987;2(8571):1316–1319.
4 Gram IT, Funkhouser E, Tabár L. The Tabár classification of mammographic parenchymal patterns. *Eur J Radiol.* 1997;24:131–136.
5 Tot T, Tabár L, Dean PB. The pressing need for better histologic-mammographic correlation of the many variations in human breast anatomy. *Virchows Arch.* 2000;437:338–344.
6 Tabár L, Dean PB, Tot T. *Teaching atlas of mammography.* 3rd ed. Stuttgart, New York:Georg Thieme Verlag; 2001.

Chapter 2

General Morphology
of Breast Lesions

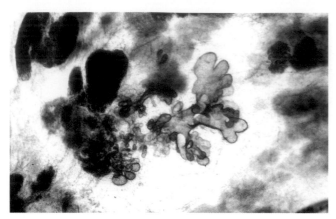

Fig. 2.**1**

Most pathologic processes in the breast originate in the terminal ductal-lobular units (TDLUs). The affected TDLUs are distended, distorted, or destroyed by the accumulation of fluid, mucin, cancer cells, necrotic debris, or calcium in the lumina of the acini and of the terminal duct or by the accumulation of collagen, glycoproteins, or stromal cells in the intralobular stroma (Fig. 2.**1**, thick-section image).

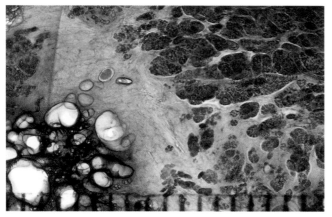

Fig. 2.**2**

If the pathologic process primarily distends and distorts the TDLU, spherical or oval lesions develop (Fig. 2.**2**, thick-section image).

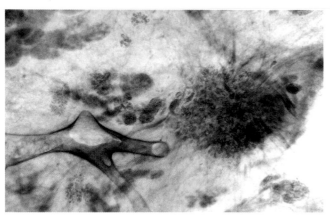

Fig. 2.**3**

If the pathologic process destroys and replaces the pre-existent TDLU, a stellate lesion may develop (Fig. 2.**3**, thick-section image).

All pathologic processes lead to a considerable enlargement of the TDLU. In neoplasia, the largest diameter of the largest invasive lesion is considered to be the *tumor size.*

As a result of distension or destruction, or both, most breast tumors are round/oval (Fig. 2.**4**) or stellate (Fig. 2.**5**).

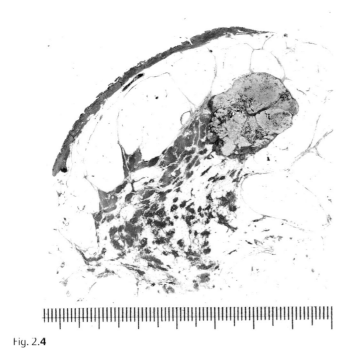

Fig. 2.**4**

Fig. 2.**5**

Fig. 2.**6**

By coalescence of the distended, distorted, and destroyed structures and invasion of the tumor into the interlobular stroma, the shape of the lesion may become increasingly complex (Fig. 2.**6**).

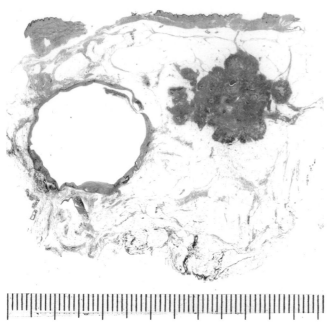

Fig. 2.**7**

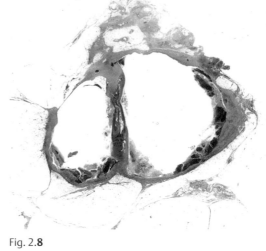

Fig. 2.**8**

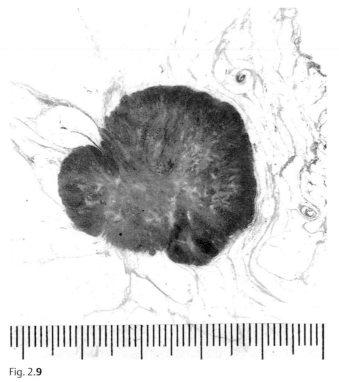

Fig. 2.**9**

Fig. 2.**10**

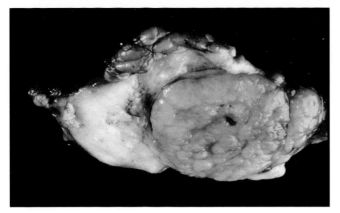

Fig. 2.**11**

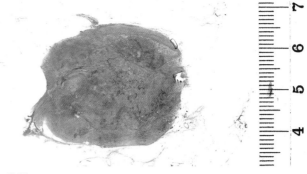

Fig. 2.**12**

The spherical/oval shape is not tumor-specific and can be seen in different pathologic processes, such as: cysts (Figs. 2.**7** and 2.**8**) and fibroadenomas; medullary (Fig. 2.**7**), mucinous (Fig. 2.**4**), and ductal carcinomas (Fig. 2.**9**); metastases in the breast (Fig. 2.**10**); and malignant mesenchymal tumors (Figs. 2.**11** and 2.**12**).

On the other hand, stellate lesions are usually carcinomatous, but may seldom be radial scars or fibrous scars (Fig. 2.**13**, thick-section image).

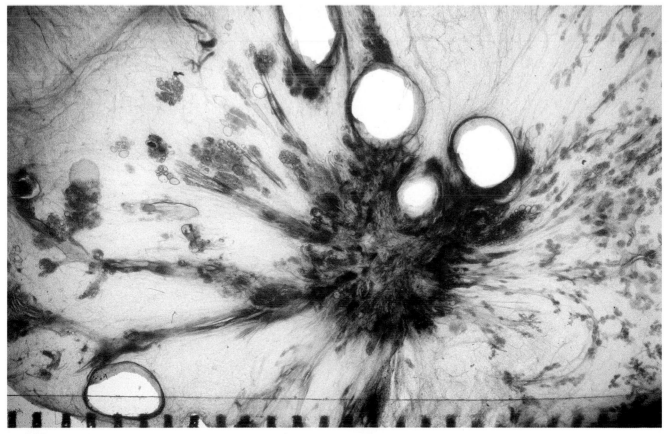

Fig. 2.**13**

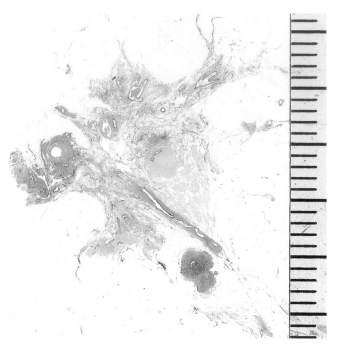

Fig. 2.**14**

If the pathologic process involves only one TDLU or a few neighboring TDLUs, a unifocal lesion develops (Fig. 2.**14**).

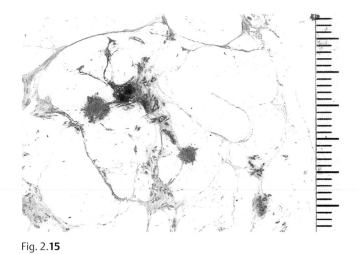

Fig. 2.**15**

If the pathologic process simultaneously involves more than one distant TDLU leaving uninvolved TDLUs in between, the lesions are considered to be multiple (multifocal) (Fig. 2.**15**).

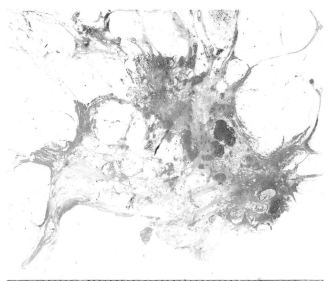

Fig. 2.**16**

When there is simultaneous involvement of a large number of TDLUs, the lesion may exhibit a diffuse growth pattern (Fig. 2.**16**).

Thus, lesions in the breast may have one of the following three distributions: solitary (unifocal), multiple (multifocal) and diffuse.

If more than one TDLU is involved, all may exhibit the same pathologic process, but often different processes are present at the same time: in situ and invasive lesions coexist, different tumor types may be present, and the tumor grade may vary considerably within same specimen. The resulting complex histologic picture is an expression of intratumoral heterogeneity (Figs. 2.17 and 2.18). Intratumoral heterogeneity may develop even in a unifocal tumor when different tumor cell clones evolve during tumor progression and dedifferentiation.

Intratumoral heterogeneity may also make the measurement of the tumor size insufficient to represent the whole lesion. The entire area of the present invasive and in situ foci has to be assessed. This parameter is referred to as the *extent of the disease*.

Fig. 2.**17**

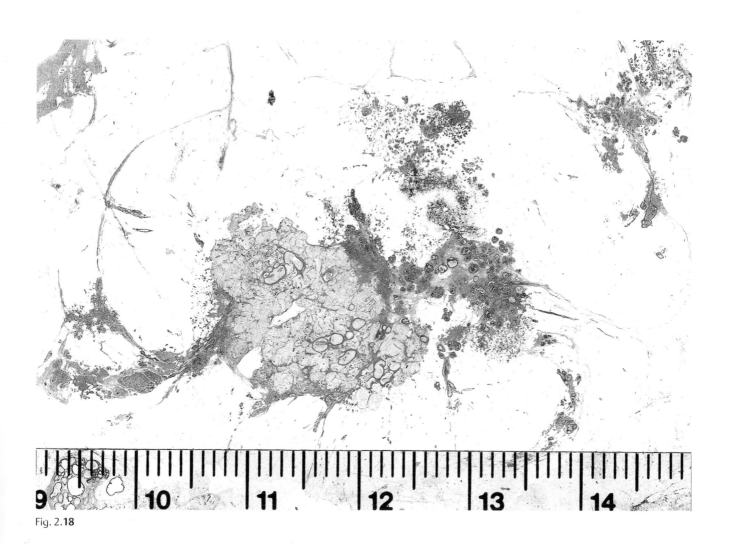

Fig. 2.**18**

The *location* of the lesions can be objectively determined by a combination of clinical, mammographic, and ultrasound parameters. To achieve uniform terminology, a horizontal plane and a vertical plane going through the nipple divide the breast into four quadrants: the upper lateral, upper medial, lower medial, and lower lateral. In addition, a fifth area of the central, retroareolar cylinder is defined (Fig. 2.**19**). By applying different orthogonal projections when imaging the breast, the radiologist can measure the distance between the lesion and the nipple. Since the location of the lesion within the breast cannot be determined solely from a histologic section, a system of marking the operative specimen is needed to provide orientation.

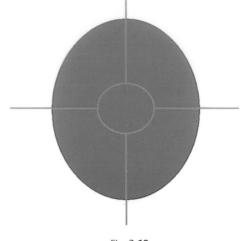

Fig. 2.**19**

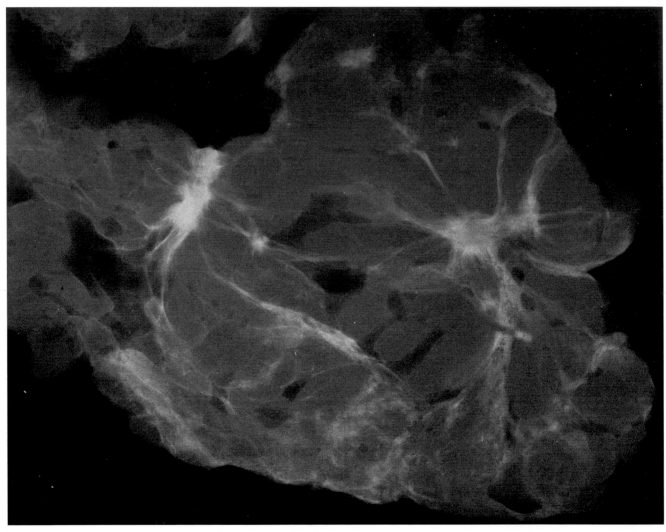

Fig. 2.**20**

Mammography and ultrasound examinations provide a good overview of the entire breast. The *size*, *extent* (the involved area), *distribution* (unifocal, multifocal, or diffuse), and *location* of the lesions are usually well seen. Even when the lesions are not seen directly on the mammogram but are detected by indirect signs–such as microcalcifications–the size, extent, distribution, and location of the lesions can still be well marked. The size, extent, and distribution of the lesions are well seen on the specimen radiograph postoperatively (Figs. 2.**20** and 2.**21**).

Histologic examination of the specimen is always necessary to further characterize the pathologic process after its size, extent, and distribution have already been indicated by the mammogram. Histologic examination should prove or rule out malignancy, delineate the in situ and the invasive components, grade and type the tumors, reveal intratumoral heterogeneity if present, and provide further morphologic–prognostic factors needed for therapy. Usually, and especially in cases of "indirect mammographic signs," the more sensitive method of histology reveals more details than the mammogram itself.

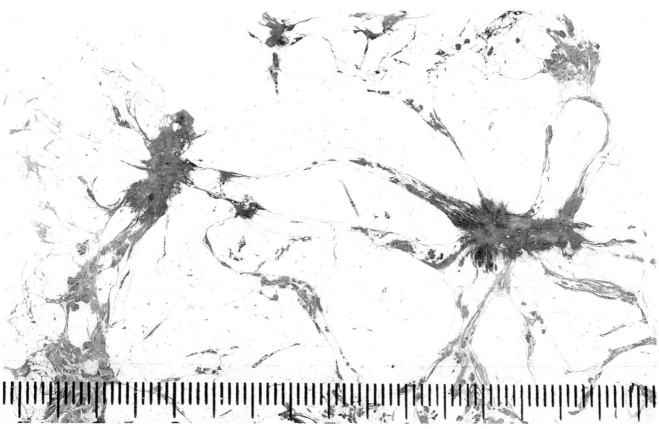

Fig. 2.**21**

Conclusions

For a successful collaboration within the breast team, radiologists, surgeons, oncologists, and pathologists must each understand the terminology used by the other members of the team. Assessment of the *size, distribution,extent*, and *location* of the lesions preoperatively and postoperatively using the mammographic–pathologic correlative approach is a prerequisite for successful collaboration. These parameters are not only important diagnostic and prognostic features; they also represent the basis for proper planning of surgical interventions and oncologic therapy.

Chapter 3

Hyperplastic Changes with and without Atypia

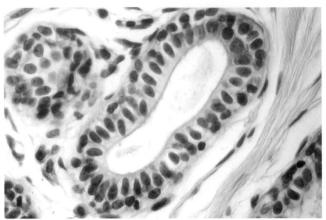

Fig. 3.**1**

The normal ducts and lobules in the breast exhibit a single layer each of epithelial and myoepithelial cells (Fig. 3.**1**).

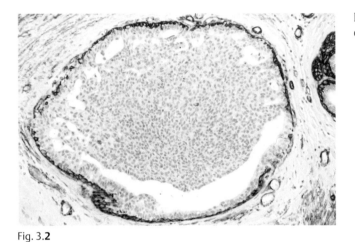

Fig. 3.**2**

In epithelial hyperplasia, more than one layer of epithelial cells is present (Fig. 3.**2**).

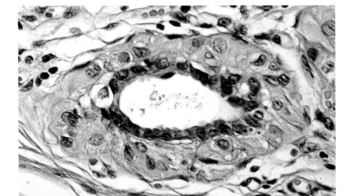

Fig. 3.**3**

In myoepithelial hyperplasia, more than one layer of myo-epithelial cells is seen (Fig. 3.**3**).

Hyperplasia may be a focal or a diffuse phenomenon involving a portion of the terminal ductal-lobular unit (TDLU), the entire TDLU, or many TDLUs and ducts.

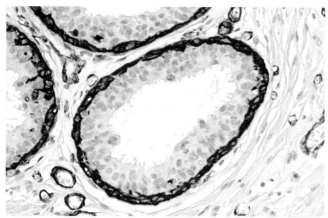

Fig. 3.**4**

Epithelial hyperplasia may result in the formation of only two to three layers of epithelial cells (Fig. 3.**4**), but often many layers of epithelial cells are present and form gland-like spaces or small papilloma-like structures ("florid" epithelial hyperplasia, Fig. 3.**5**).

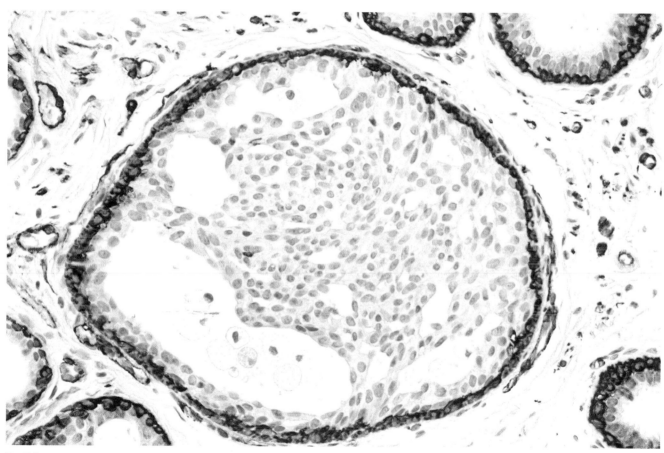

Fig. 3.**5**

Neoplasia may also result in several layers of epithelial cells within the ducts and acini. Hyperplasia and neoplasia can be differentiated on the basis of their cellular and architectural characteristics.

Cellular Characteristics

Hyperplasia is a benign proliferation of several cell clones resulting in a *polymorphous population of small cells* (Fig. 3.**6**).

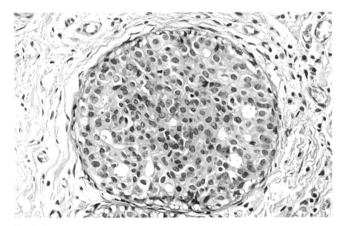

Fig. 3.**6**

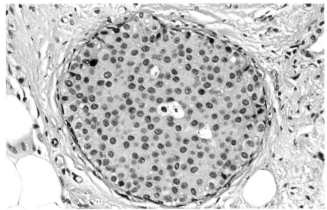

Fig. 3.**7**

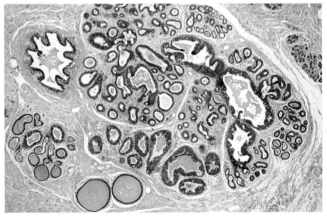

Fig. 3.**8**

Low-grade malignant epithelial cells appear as a monoclonal, *monomorphous population of small cells* (Fig. 3.**7**). These cells also give rise to several layers of cells within the ducts and lobules, resembling hyperplasia, and they may even appear within epithelial hyperplasia, partly taking over the structures. If only a portion of the TDLU is replaced by this monomorphous cell population, the lesion is called atypical ductal hyperplasia (ADH) (Fig. 3.**8**). If the entire TDLU is filled by the monomorphous small cells, the lesion is considered to be ductal carcinoma in situ (DCIS) grade I. ADH differs from DCIS grade I through extent and distribution, not through cellular features.

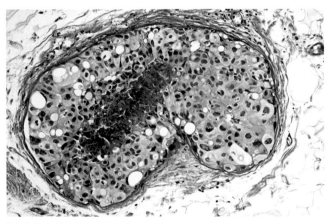

Fig. 3.**9**

During the evolution of DCIS, different cell clones may appear within the initially monoclonal tumor cell population leading to a multiclonal malignant cell population. These lesions are grade II or grade III DCIS and consist of *a population of large polymorphous cells* (Fig. 3.**9**).

Architectural Features

The gland-like structures in hyperplasia are irregular, often slit-like, and of different sizes and shapes (Fig. 3.**10**). They become partly uniform and more "rigid" in ADH (Fig. 3.**11**), and regular and uniformly round or oval throughout the whole lesion in DCIS (Fig. 3.**12**).

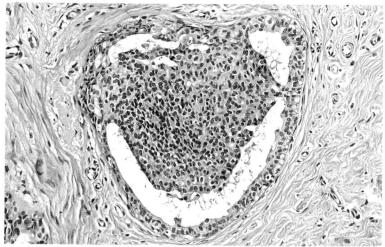

Fig. 3.**10**

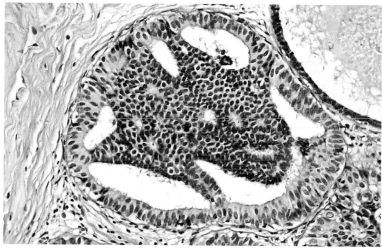

Fig. 3.**11**

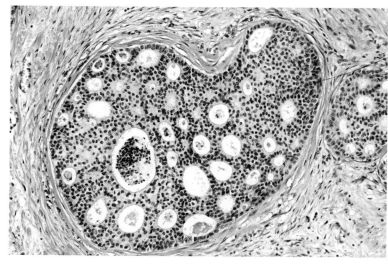

Fig. 3.**12**

An additional differential diagnostic feature is the polarity of the cells within the "bridges." In hyperplasia the cell nuclei are usually longitudinally oriented (Fig. 3.13), whereas in ADH and DCIS the cell nuclei are perpendicular relative to the axis of the bridges (Fig. 3.14).

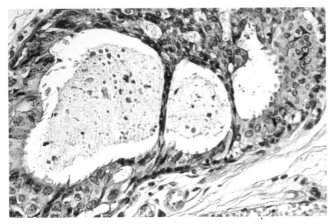

Fig. 3.13

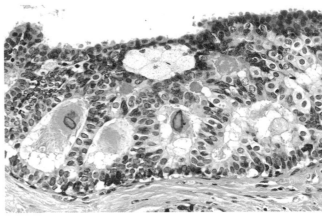

Fig. 3.14

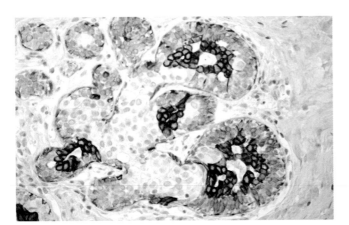

Fig. 3.15

As a polyclonal cell population, epithelial cells in hyperplasia often express antigens otherwise typical of myoepithelium (e.g., cytokeratin 5–6). These antigens are absent from the cells in ADH and DCIS. Figures 3.15 and 3.16 show a TDLU partly filled with structures of epithelial hyperplasia (stained positively for cytokeratin 5–6) and partly with unstained malignant cells.

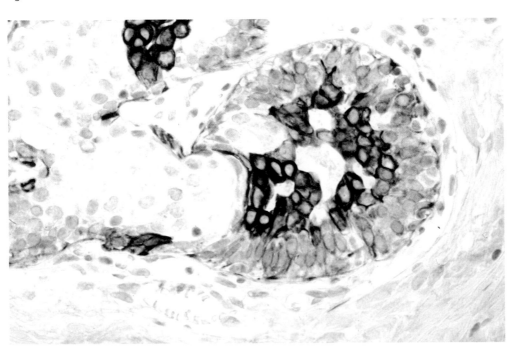

Fig. 3.16

Summary

Hyperplasia:	Polymorphous population of small cells Irregular gland-like spaces Longitudinally oriented nuclei in the bridges Myoepithelial antigens often expressed No restrictions on extent and distribution
DCIS grade I:	Monomorphous population of small cells Regular, "rigid" gland-like structures Perpendicularly oriented nuclei in the bridges Myoepithelial antigens usually absent No restrictions on extent and distribution
ADH:	Features of DCIS grade I, with restrictions on extent and distribution TDLU is only partly involved No more than two TDLUs are involved A single lesion is not larger than 2 mm

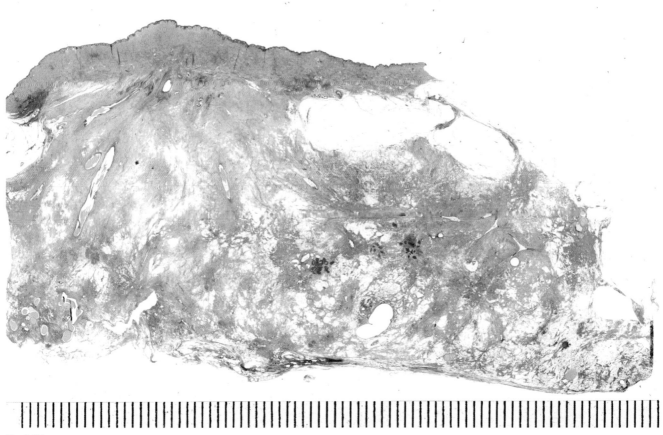

Fig. 3.**17**

Figure 3.**17** shows a borderline case between ADH and DCIS grade I: two TDLUs are involved, both are 2 mm in size.

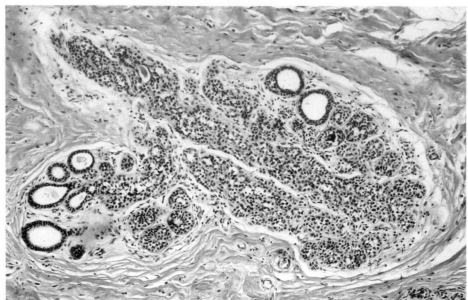

Fig. 3.**18**

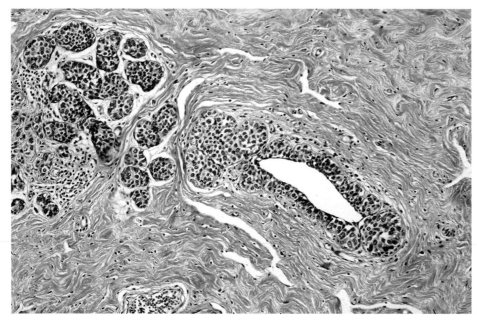

Fig. 3.**19**

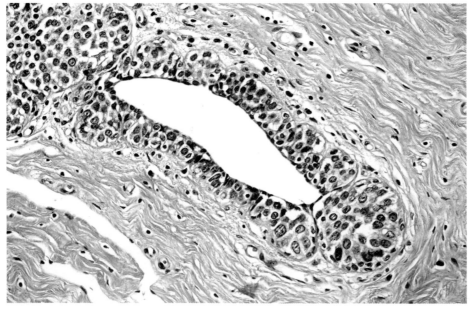

Fig. 3.**20**

Hyperplasia may be seen in the acini as well as in the ducts. Another phenomenon is the appearance of small, loosely packed cells that fill the lumina of the acini within the lobules. These cells often contain a small intracytoplasmic vacuole that pushes the nucleus aside. The cells have the same appearance as the cells of invasive lobular carcinoma (see Chapter 5). If most of the acini within the lobules are filled with these cells, the lesion is *lobular carcinoma in situ (LCIS)* (Fig. 3.**19**). The cells of LCIS may spread into the terminal duct in the form of small intraepithelial nests ("pagetoid spread") (Fig. 3.**20**). If only some acini are filled while the others have an open lumen, the lesion is *atypical lobular hyperplasia (ALH)* (Fig. 3.**18**).

All of these lesions–hyperplasia, atypical hyperplasia, and carcinoma in situ–have their origins in the TDLU. Designating them as "ductal" or "lobular" is a more traditional way of discriminating two genetically and phenotypically different types of breast tumors: one consisting of cohesively packed cells building gland-like and papillary structures and the other consisting of loosely packed dispersed cells. Florid epithelial hyperplasia, ADH, and LCIS are "marker lesions" of an increased risk of developing invasive carcinomas in both breasts. These marker lesions are often multifocal and bilateral.

Conclusions

Florid epithelial hyperplasia, atypical ductal hyperplasia, atypical lobular hyperplasia, and ductal carcinoma in situ grade I are "borderline" proliferative lesions that represent a marker of increased risk of subsequent development of invasive (usually low-grade) carcinomas. Although they are morphologically similar, they can be classified properly in most cases on the basis of established criteria.

References

1. Page DL, Dupont WD. Premalignant conditions and markers of elevated risk in the breast and their management. *Surg Clin North Am.* 1990;70:835–851.
2. Pinder SE, Ellis IO. Atypical ductal hyperplasia, ductal carcinoma in situ and in situ atypical apocrine proliferations of the breast. *Curr Diagn Pathol.* 1996;3:235–242.
3. Otterbach F, et al. Cytokeratin 5/6 immunohistochemistry assists the differential diagnosis of atypical proliferations of the breast. *Histopathology.* 2000;37:232–240.

Chapter 4

Ductal Carcinoma In Situ (DCIS)

Carcinoma in situ is a malignant tumor growing in spaces surrounded by an intact basement membrane.

These spaces are either preformed, pre-existing ducts or lobules, or newly formed acini, lobules, or ducts (Fig. 4.1).

The diagnostic criteria for carcinoma in situ are:

– intact basement membrane (Fig. 4.2)

– malignant cells not invading through the basement membrane

Malignancy of the tumor cells can be illustrated immunohistochemically –for example, by staining on oncogene c-erbB-2 (Fig. 4.3).

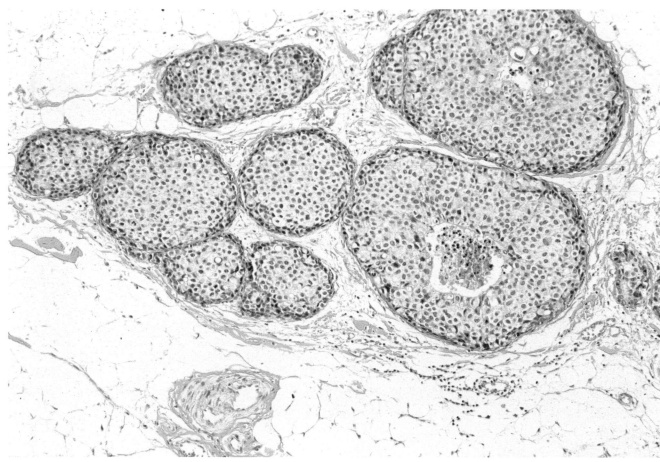

Fig. 4.1

The criterion of an intact basement membrane (Fig. 4.4, collagen IV stain) is more accurate for determining the invasiveness of breast carcinoma because the myoepithelial cell layer may be discontinuous or focally absent (Fig. 4.5, smooth muscle actin stain).

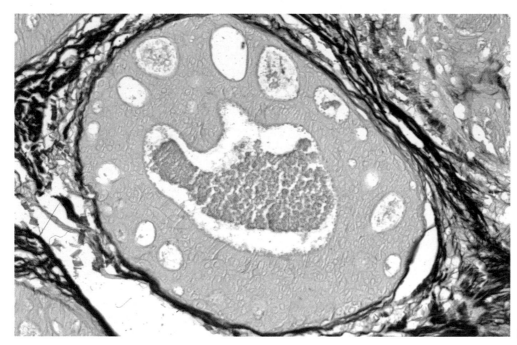

Fig. 4.**2**

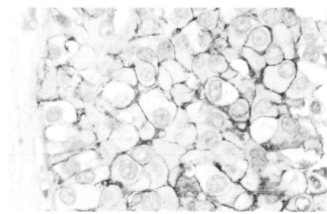

Fig. 4.**3**

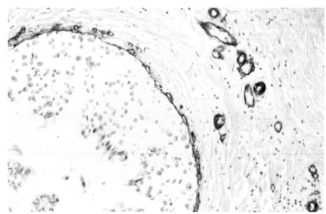

Fig. 4.**4**

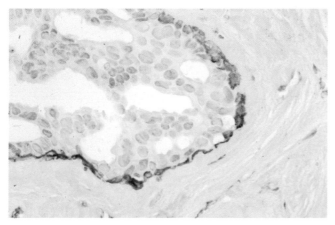

Fig. 4.**5**

As with almost all pathologic processes in the breast, ductal carcinoma in situ (DCIS) and lobular carcinoma in situ (LCIS) initially develop in a lobule. The word "ductal" indicates a tissue differentiation other than "lobular." "Ductal differentiation" means that the tumor cells are larger and more cohesive with a tendency to form gland-like or papillary structures. LCIS, on the other hand, contains smaller cells, often with a cytoplasmic vacuole; these cells are less cohesive and never form gland-like or papillary structures (see also Chapter 3). These characteristics allow the pathologist to delineate the two basic types of carcinoma in situ, DCIS and LCIS, in the vast majority of cases. However, DCIS itself is a heterogeneous disease that needs to be further stratified by grading and subtyping.

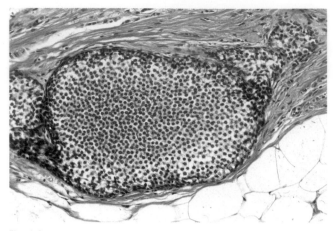

Fig. 4.**6**

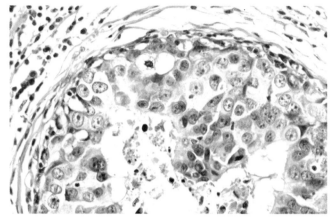

Fig. 4.**7**

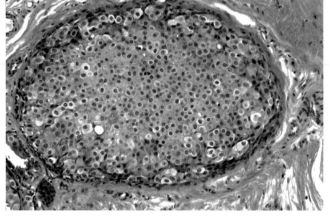

Fig. 4.**8**

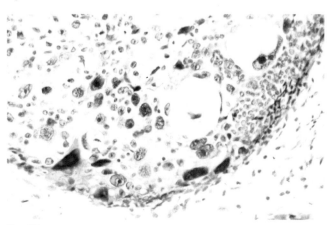

Fig. 4.**9**

When grading DCIS, the most important histopathologic prognostic factor is the *nuclear grade*, as follows:

Low nuclear grade: monomorphous, small nuclei, no or very few regular mitoses, no or few apoptotic bodies (Fig. 4.**6**). The nuclei are usually diploid and estrogen-receptor positive.

High nuclear grade: polymorphous, large nuclei with high mitotic rate and many apoptotic bodies (Fig. 4.**7**). Irregular mitoses can be present. The nuclei are usually aneuploid and estrogen-receptor negative.

Intermediate nuclear grade: somewhat enlarged and somewhat polymorphous nuclei with few mitoses and few apoptotic bodies (Fig. 4.**8**).

The nuclear grade may vary considerably in the same DCIS (Fig. 4.**9**). In these cases, the use of the highest nuclear grade is recommended.

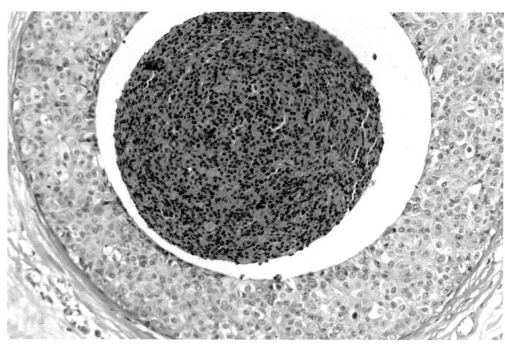

Fig. 4.**10**

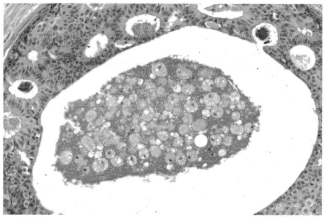

Fig. 4.**11**

The second most important histopathologic prognostic factor in grading DCIS is the presence or absence of *central necrosis* in the lumen of the ducts and acini. This necrosis is the result of cell death, as indicated by the presence of apoptotic nuclear fragments in the necrotic debris (Fig. 4.**10**). Secretion in the lumen of the ducts with DCIS, which often contain degenerated cells (Fig. 4.**11**), must be recognized as not representing necrosis.

A simple practical grading system of DCIS is recommended, as follows:

DCIS grade I: low nuclear grade without central necrosis

DCIS grade II: low nuclear grade with central necrosis, or intermediate nuclear grade (with or without central necrosis)

DCIS grade III: high nuclear grade (with or without central necrosis)

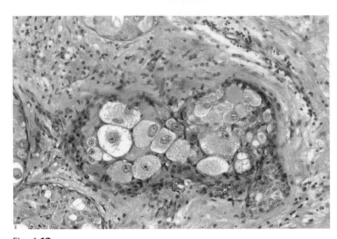

Fig. 4.**12**

The tumor cells of DCIS may express phenotypic variations enabling the recognition of DCIS subtypes, such as:

– apocrine DCIS (Fig. 4.**12**)

– endocrine DCIS (Fig. 4.**13**)

– clear-cell DCIS (Fig. 4.**14**)

– signet-ring cell DCIS (Fig. 4.**15**)

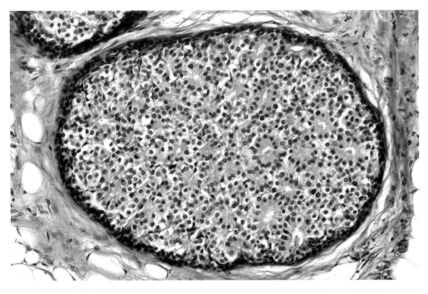

Fig. 4.**13**

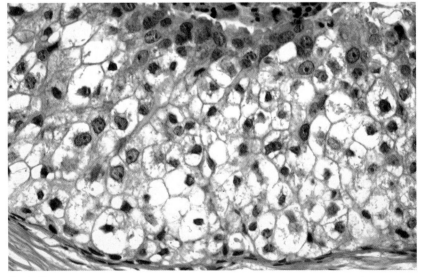

Fig. 4.**14**

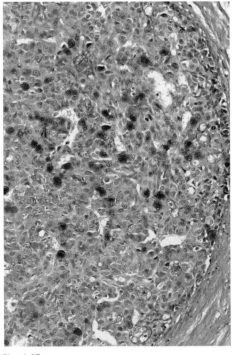

Fig. 4.**15**

This subtyping, though morphologically simple and straightforward, has only minimal clinical value.

The growth pattern of DCIS is important to the histologist for the differential diagnosis of DCIS, benign hyperplasia, atypical ductal hyperplasia, and LCIS.

The patterns are:

– micropapillary DCIS (Fig. 4.**16**)
– cribriform DCIS (Fig. 4.**17**)
– solid DCIS (Fig. 4.**18**)
– clinging DCIS (Fig. 4.**19**)

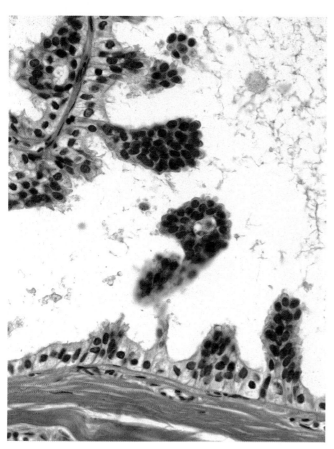

Fig. 4.**16**

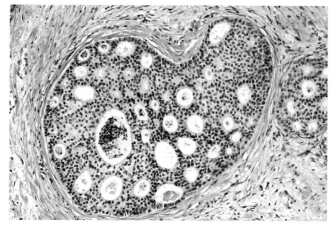

Fig. 4.**17**

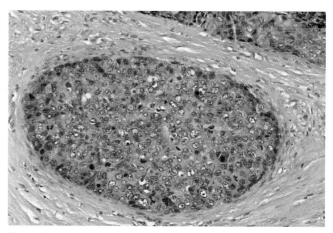

Fig. 4.**18**

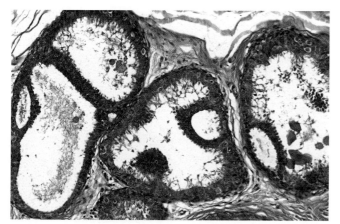

Fig. 4.**19**

The growth pattern may influence the mammographic appearance of DCIS as well as the clinical picture. However, the growth pattern itself has no prognostic value, because every pattern can be associated with low, intermediate, and high nuclear grade and may or may not show central necrosis.

The central necrotic material often becomes dystrophically calcified forming large, irregular, elongated, or triangular and frequently quite extensive *amorphous microcalcifications* (Figs. 4.**20** and 4.**21**), which can be readily visualized on the mammogram.

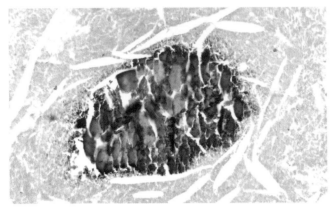

Fig. 4.**20**

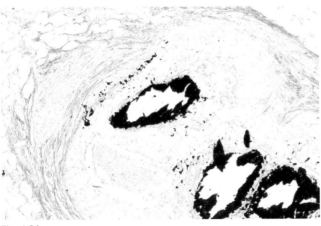

Fig. 4.**21**

The secretions in the lumen of DCIS grade I may calcify and form *psammoma bodies* (Fig. 4.**24**), which are small and laminated and are detectable on the mammogram as *powdery microcalcifications* only when numerous (Fig. 4.**25**).

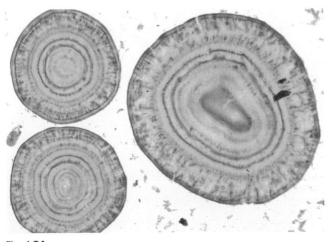

Fig. 4.**24**

The amorphous calcifications of DCIS tend to gradually fill the ducts and appear as long, branching calcifications on the mammogram, the so-called *casting type calcifications* (Fig. 4.**22**). If the DCIS fills a dilated lobule, the calcifications may appear as triangular or *"broken needle type"* ("crushed-stone–like") (Fig. 4.**23**) often in clusters.

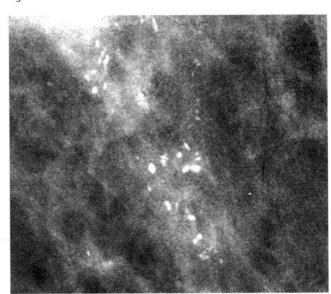

Fig. 4.**22**

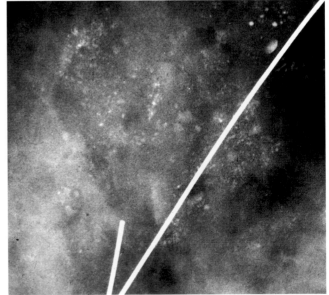

Fig. 4.**23**

Fig. 4.**25**

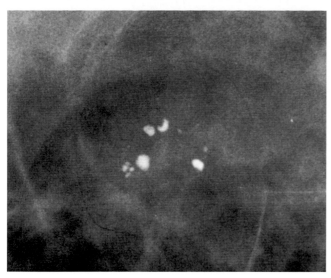

Fig. 4.**26**

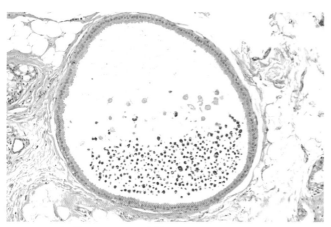

Fig. 4.**27**

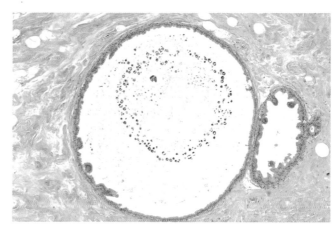

Fig. 4.**28**

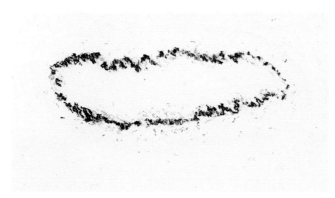

Fig. 4.**29**

Microcalcifications appear in many benign conditions in the breast. In fibrocystic change, the microcalcifications are often teacup-like or annular (Figs. 4.**26**–4.**28**). While the casting type of microcalcifications is almost specific for DCIS, clusters of the broken-needle type of calcifications may appear in fibroadenomas, fibrocystic change, or papillomas. Powdery microcalcifications are often seen in sclerosing adenosis. Calcified arteries typically appear as double linear calcifications (Fig. 4.**29**).

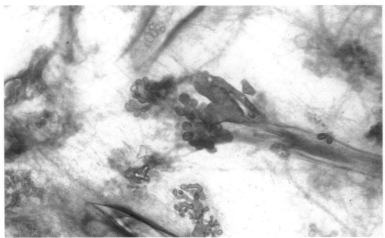

Fig. 4.**30**

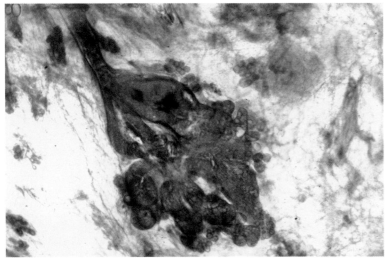

Fig. 4.**31**

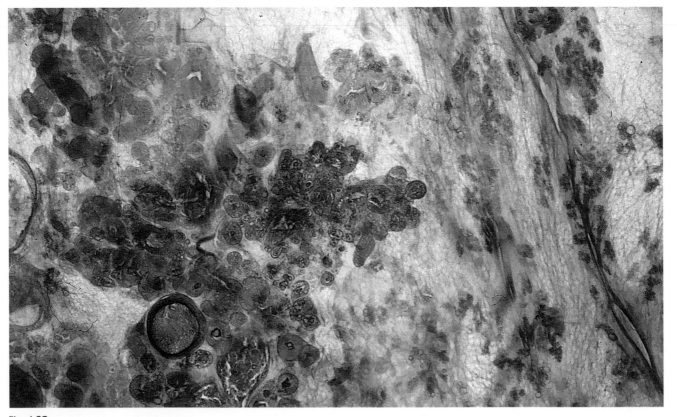

Fig. 4.**32**

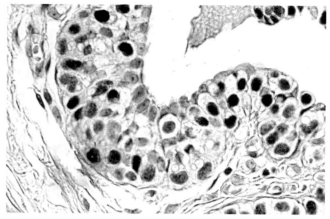

Fig. 4.**33**

As mentioned previously, DCIS initially develops in one or several terminal ductal-lobular units (TDLUs) (Fig. 4.**30**, thick-section image). In less aggressive cases of DCIS, the tumor does not leave the TDLU but causes dilatation and distortion of the affected TDLU (Figs. 4.**31** and 4.**32**, thick-section images).

Like the cells of LCIS, the tumor cells of DCIS may spread in the form of subepithelial cell groups in the terminal and subsegmental ducts –a phenomenon called "pagetoid spread" (Fig. 4.**33**) (see also Chapter 3).

In more aggressive cases of DCIS, the tumor leaves the TDLU and engages the neighboring ducts and TDLUs growing into the lumen of the normal acini (the so-called cancerization of the lobules) (Figs. 4.**34** and 4.**35**).

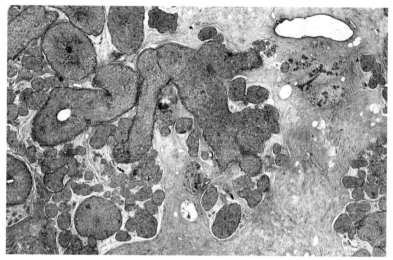

Fig. 4.**34**

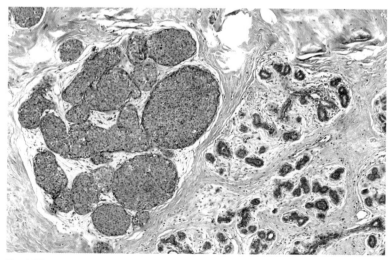

Fig. 4.**35**

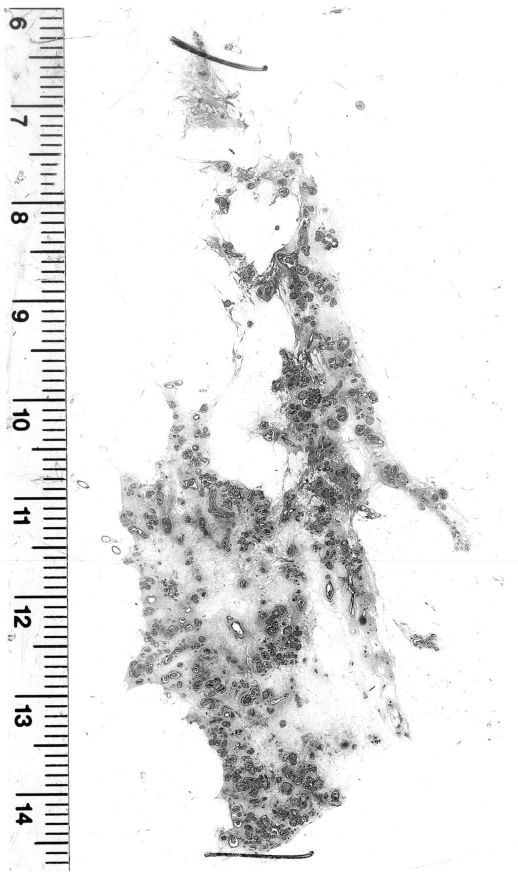

Fig. 4.**36**

Figure 4.**36** shows a case of DCIS grade III with more ducts in the area of the tumor as compared with the area of the remaining normal breast. In some very aggressive cases, the tumor may form new duct-like structures as a consequence of tumor extension. These structures are also surrounded by the basement membrane. Periductal lymphocytic infiltration (Figs. 4.**37** and 4.**38**) and periductal tenascin accumulation (Figs. 4.**39** and 4.**40**) may represent an indirect sign of "duct neogenesis."

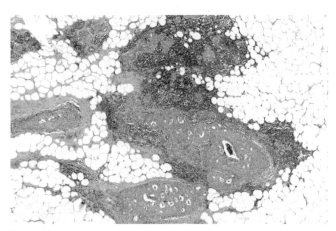

Fig. 4.**37**

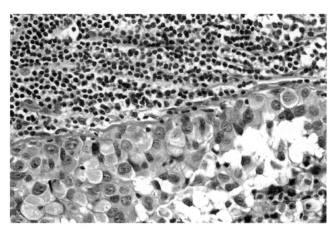

Fig. 4.**38**

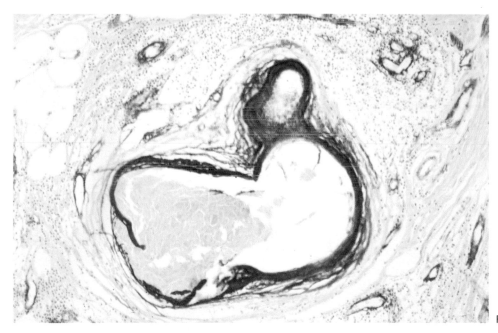

Fig. 4.**39**

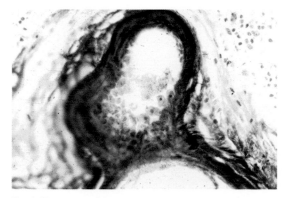

Fig. 4.**40**

The prognostically different categories of DCIS differ from each other not only in histologic grade (I, II, and III), but also in their *extent* and *distribution*. Because tumor size is defined by the largest diameter of the largest invasive focus, DCIS lacks this parameter.

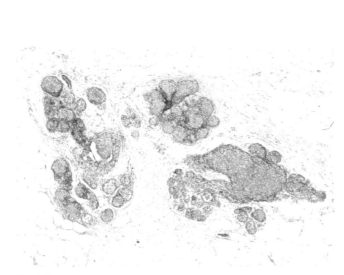

Fig. 4.**41**

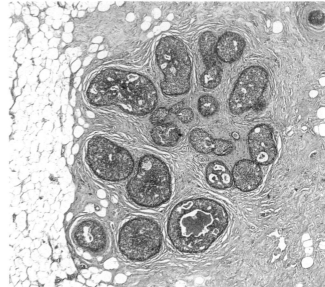

Fig. 4.**43**

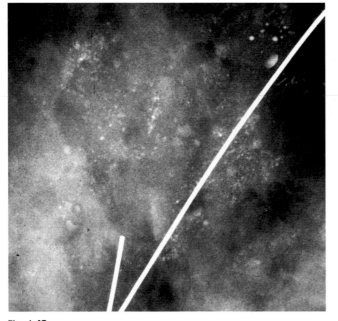

Fig. 4.**42**

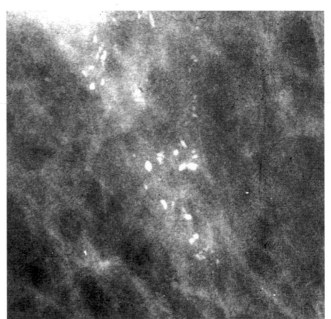

Fig. 4.**44**

DCIS grade I typically appears as multiple, somewhat dilated and distorted lobules filled with cancer cells (Fig. 4.**41**). It may contain psammoma-body–like microcalcifications. The typical mammographic appearance in these cases is the presence of powdery microcalcifications (Fig. 4.**42**). This grade of DCIS may be *extensive and multifocal.*

DCIS grade II usually grows in an extremely dilated TDLU (Fig. 4.**43**). Central necrosis is often present with or without microcalcifications. The calcifications are amorphous and the "broken-needle type" (Fig. 4.**44**). This DCIS is of *limited extent, often unifocal* or less significantly multifocal.

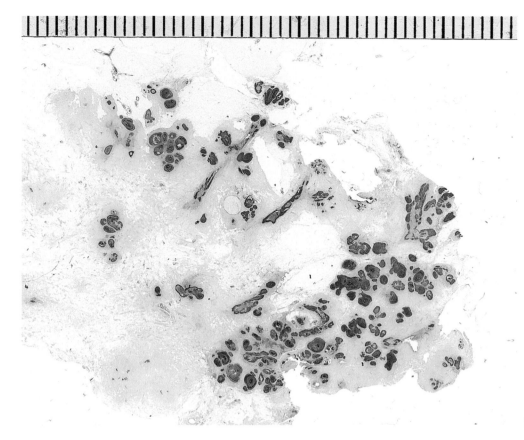

Fig. 4.**45**

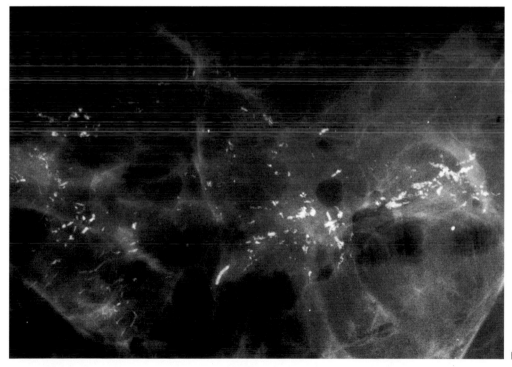

Fig. 4.**46**

DCIS grade III leaves the TDLU at an early stage of development and has the potential both to fill preformed ducts and lobules as well as to form new ducts (Fig. 4.**45**). This grade of DCIS often contains "casting type" microcalcifications (Fig. 4.**46**). DCIS grade III is often *extensive, diffuse,* and aggressive.

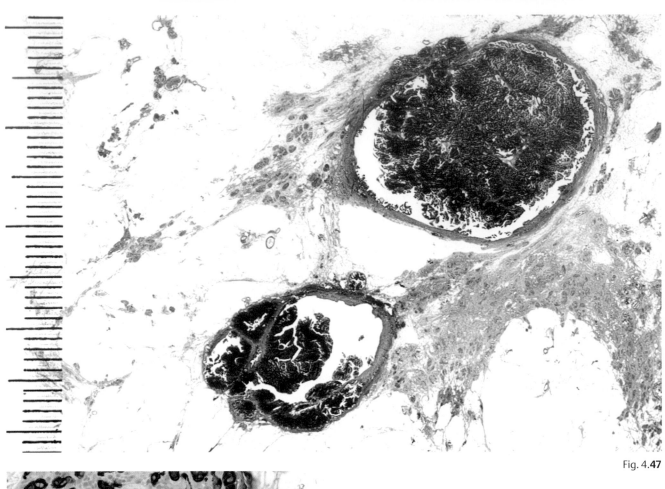

Fig. 4.**47**

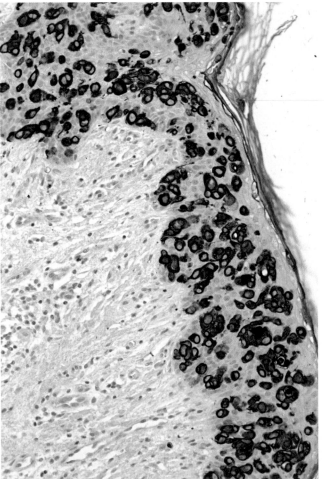

Fig. 4.**48**

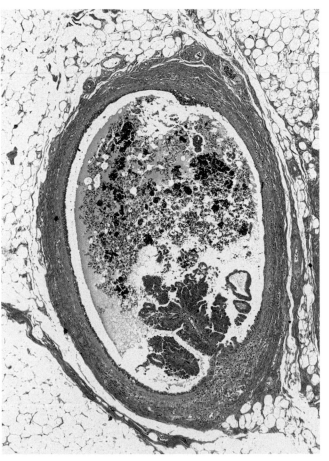

Fig. 4.**49**

Most cases of DCIS are nonpalpable and asymptomatic and are detected by finding microcalcifications at mammographic screening. However, about 20% of cases of DCIS, the so-called special types, are clinically detectable displaying:

- a palpable cystic tumor (intracystic papillary carcinoma, Fig. 4.**47**) (see also Chapter 6)

- a chronic, eczema-like skin lesion in the region of the nipple/areola (Paget disease, Fig. 4.**48**, cytokeratin CAM 5,2 staining)

- nipple discharge (intraductal papilloma with DCIS, see Chapter 6, or the so-called apocrine papillary DCIS, Fig. 4.**49**)

- a palpable stellate lesion on the mammogram (so-called tumor-forming DCIS, Figs. 4.**50** and 4.**51**)

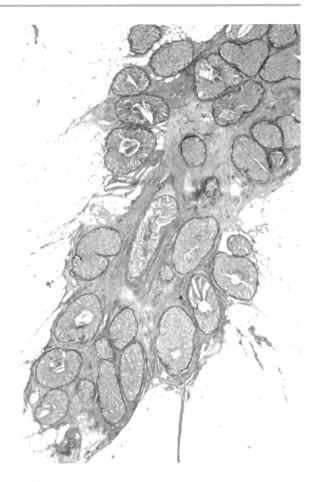

Fig. 4.**51**

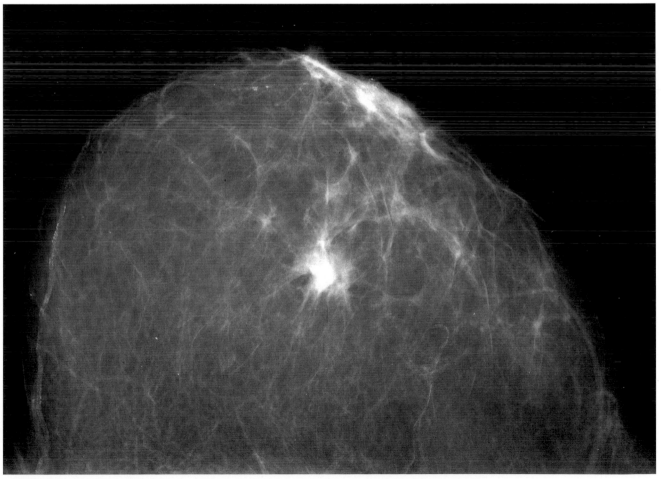

Fig. 4.**50**

Unlike florid epithelial hyperplasia, LCIS, and atypical ductal hyperplasia (ADH), which are marker lesions for an increased risk of developing invasive cancer in both breasts, DCIS grade I is a marker for an increased risk of developing invasive cancer in the same breast after a period of several years. The prognosis in these cases is very good.

DCIS grade III is often a highly aggressive lesion with recurrences even after a seemingly radical excision. Extensive invasive recurrences may develop over a short period. Even if the invasive component is microscopic or undetectable, the prognosis may be unfavorable.

The prognosis of DCIS grade II is intermediate.

The special types of DCIS generally have a good prognosis, with the exception of Paget disease, which is usually a grade III lesion.

Conclusions

DCIS is a heterogeneous group of diseases that varies in cell type, growth pattern, presence of necrosis, nuclear grade, and extent and distribution.

Most DCIS cases are detected on the basis of microcalcifications seen on the mammogram. By assessing the type, distribution, and extent of the microcalcifications, the skillful radiologist can differentiate benign microcalcifications from microcalcifications that are suspicious for malignancy.

The most important role of the pathologist in making the diagnosis of DCIS is correct classification, especially recognizing the aggressive forms that need immediate therapeutic intervention and careful follow-up.

For a successful pathologic work-up, it is essential to:

- correlate the histologic and mammographic findings
- use a simple and reproducible grading system
- use the large-section technique because DCIS often extends beyond the area of the microcalcifications

References

1   Faverly DRG, Burgers L, Bult P, Holland R. Three dimensional imaging of mammary ductal carcinoma in situ: clinical implications. *Sem Diagn Path.* 1994;11(3):193–198.
2   Consensus conference on the classification of ductal carcinoma in situ. *Hum Pathol.* 1997;28(11):1221–1225.
3   Shoker BS, Sloane JP. DCIS grading schemes and clinical implications. *Histopathology.* 1999;35:393–400.
4   Silverstein MJ, Lagios MD, Craig PH, et al. A prognostic index for ductal carcinoma in situ of the breast. *Cancer.* 1996;77:2267–2274.

Chapter 5

The Most Common Types of Invasive Breast Carcinoma

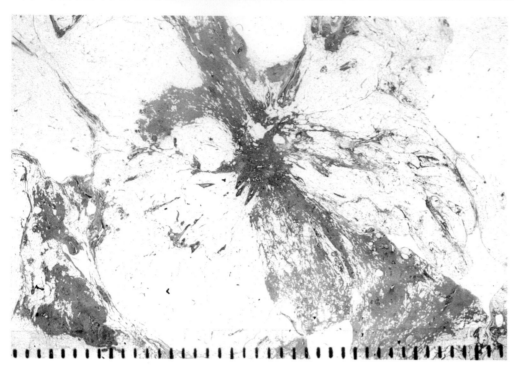

Fig. 5.**1**

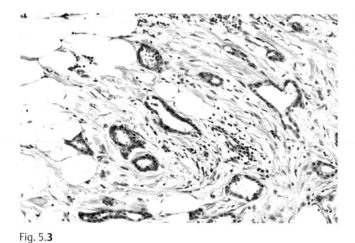

Fig. 5.**3**

Tubular carcinoma is usually a slow-growing, stellate tumor with stromal desmoplasia (Fig. 5.**1**). The typical mammographic appearance is a small stellate density with a central tumor mass ("white star") (Fig. 5.**2**).

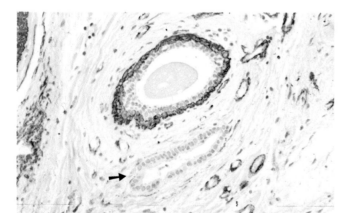

Fig. 5.**4**

Diagnostic Criteria

More than 90% of the tumor has tubular structures, which are

- angulated and irregular (Fig. 5.**3**)
- composed of only one thin layer of epithelial cells, which means
- absence of myoepithelium (Fig. 5.**4**, arrow).

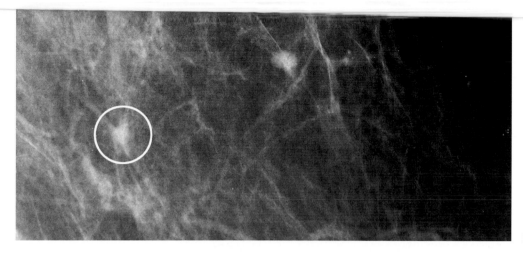

Fig. 5.**2**

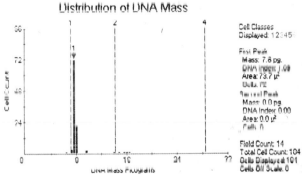

Fig 5.**5**

Tubular carcinoma is usually small and of limited extent, but it may be multifocal. Structures of ductal carcinoma in situ (DCIS) grade I are regularly present in the tumor. Tubular carcinoma is regularly diploid (Fig. 5.**5**), estrogen receptor positive (Fig. 5.**6**), and has an excellent prognosis.

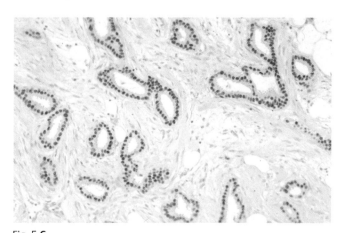

Fig. 5.**6**

Differential Diagnosis

1. Radial scar (see also Chapter 6):

   – not palpable
   – typical mammographic picture of a "black star"
   – presence of myoepithelium

2. Microglandular adenosis:
   – regular, round glands (absence of lobulocentricity and myoepithelium)

3. Invasive ductal carcinoma not otherwise specified (NOS):

   – contains less than 90% tubular structures

Mucinous carcinoma is a mucin-producing, slow-growing, tumor with a favorable prognosis. Mammographically, it usually appears as a circular – oval, ill-defined, low-density tumor mass (Fig. 5.7).

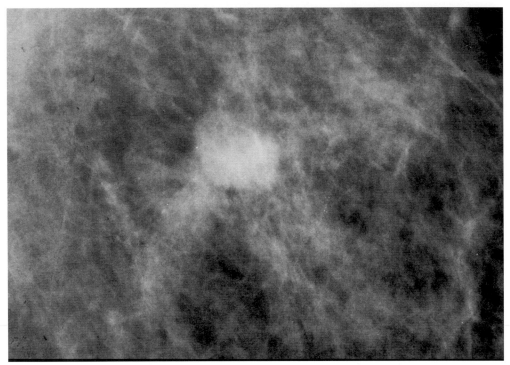

Fig. 5.**7**

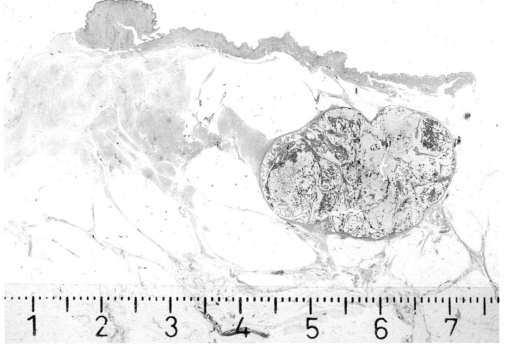

Fig. 5.**8**

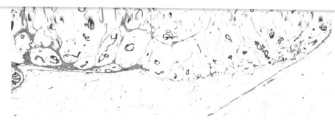

Fig. 5.**9**

A tumor fulfilling these criteria has an excellent prognosis. However, mucinous carcinoma often exhibits obvious intratumoral heterogeneity (see Chapter 10, case 1), which may have prognostic implications.

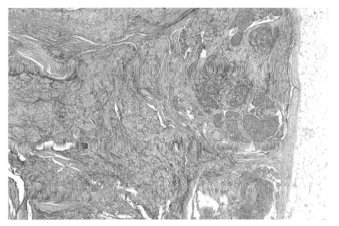

Fig. 5.**10**

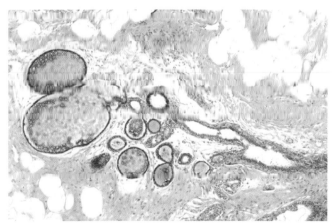

Fig. 5.**11**

Differential Diagnosis

1. Mucin containing lobules, dilated ducts, mucocele (Fig. 5.**11**), and mucinous DCIS (Fig. 5.**12**).

2. Ductal carcinoma with mucinous component:

   - poorly circumscribed, often stellate
   - more cellular
   - often less well-differentiated tumor cells

Ductal carcinomas with a mucinous component do not share the favorable prognosis of purely mucinous carcinomas.

3. Invasive micropapillary carcinoma (see Chapter 6).

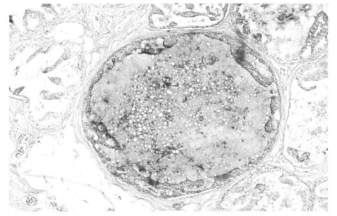

Fig. 5.**12**

Medullary carcinoma is usually a rapidly growing, round or oval, well-circumscribed tumor appearing in younger patients. Mammographically or ultrasonographically (Fig. 5.13), a circumscribed, solid, round or oval density is observed.

Macroscopically and histologically the tumor is well-circumscribed, relatively soft, and often lobulated (Fig. 5.14).

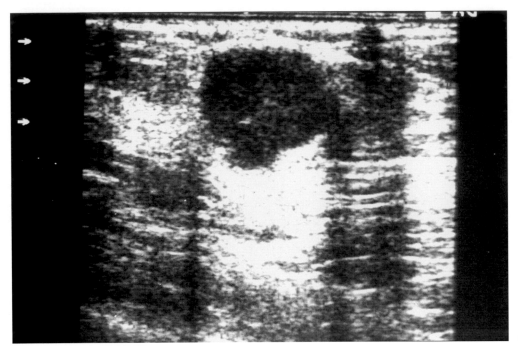

Fig. 5.**13**

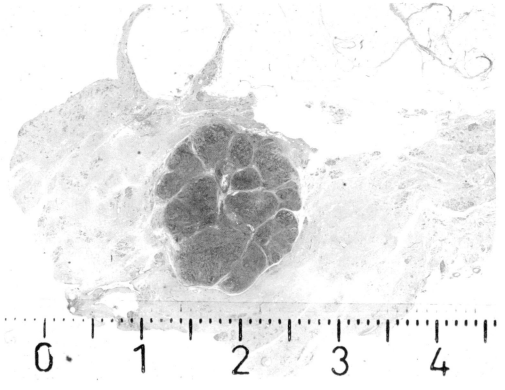

Fig. 5.**14**

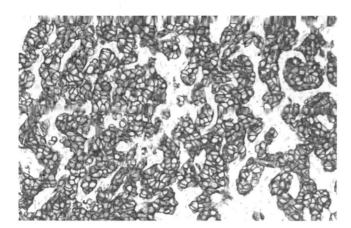

Fig. 5.**15**

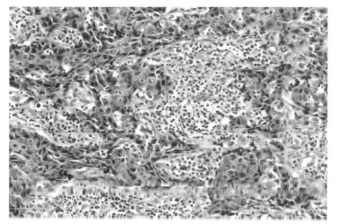

Fig. 5.**16**

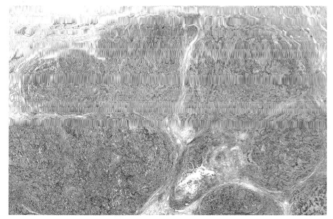

Fig. 5.**17**

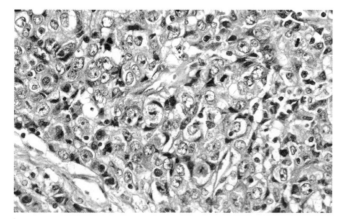

Fig. 5.**18**

Diagnostic Criteria

- Syncytial growth pattern (Fig. 5.**15**)
- Intensive lymphoplasmacytic infiltrate in the stroma (Fig. 5.**16**)
- Non-infiltrating ("pushing") tumor border (Fig. 5.**17**)
- Highly atypical tumor cells (Fig. 5.**18**)

In situ component and central fibrosis are not features of this tumor.

Tumors with all four criteria are "typical medullary carcinomas" and have a somewhat more favorable prognosis when compared with ductal carcinomas of the same size and grade. "Atypical medullary carcinomas" with only some medullary features (e.g., infiltrating tumor border as in Fig. 5.**19**) share an unfavorable prognosis with their ductal counterparts.

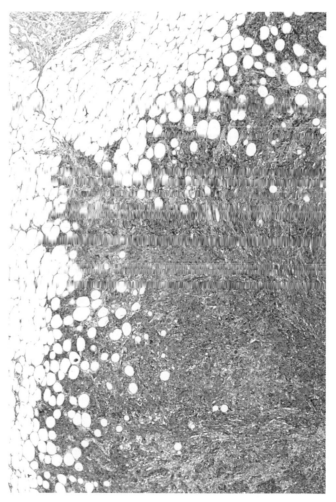

Fig. 5.**19**

Differential Diagnosis

1. Fibroadenoma (see Chapter 6).

Invasive lobular carcinomas are a heterogeneous group of tumors.

Diagnostic Criteria

- Cell files, one or two cells thick (Fig. 5.**20**) and/or
- small, monomorphous tumor cells, often with intracytoplasmic vacuoles (Fig. 5.**21**).

The criteria have alternative characteristics: tumors composed of cell files classify as lobular even if the tumor cells are larger, more polymorphous, and lacking vacuolization ("pleomorphic variant of lobular breast carcinoma," Figs. 5.**22** and 5.**29**). The tumor cells may also exhibit phenotypic variations such as a histiocytoid (Fig. 5.**23**) or a signet-ring (Fig. 5.**24**) appearance.

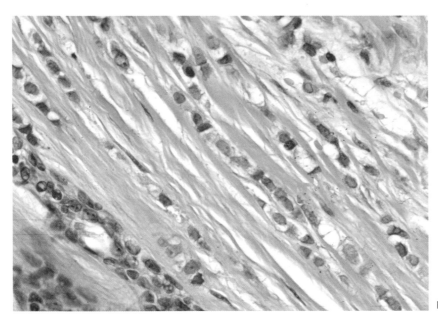

Fig. 5.**20**

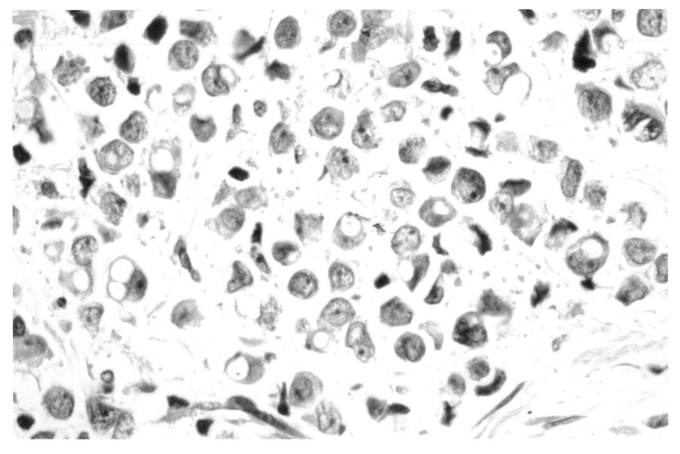

Fig. 5.**21**

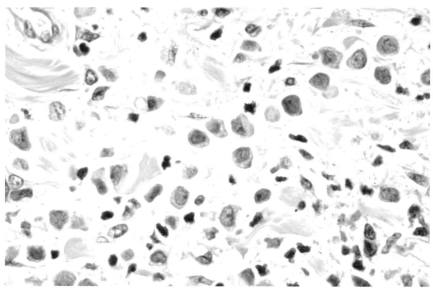

Fig. 5.**22**

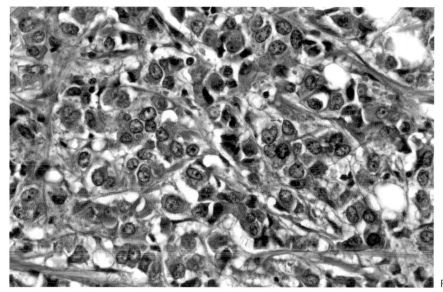

Fig. 5.**23**

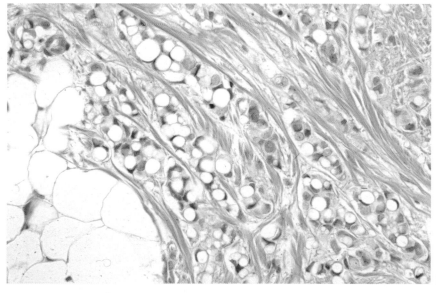

Fig. 5.**24**

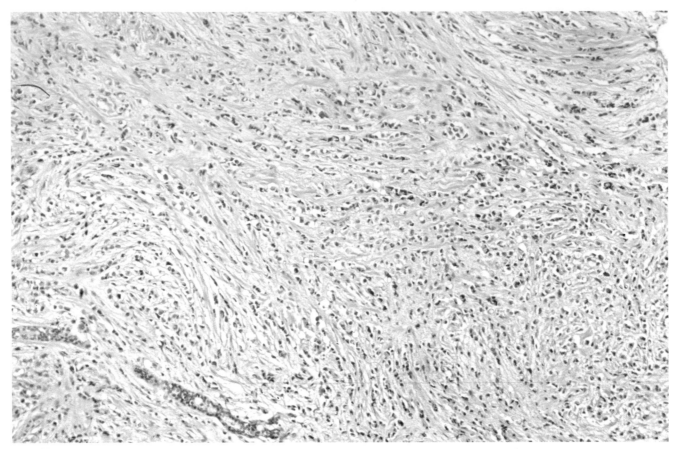

Fig. 5.**25**

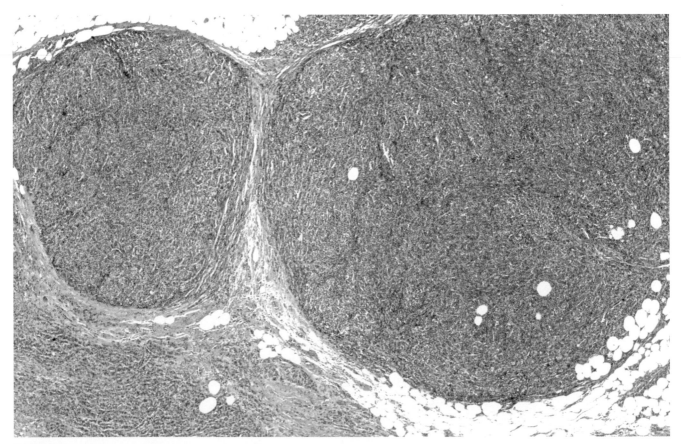

Fig. 5.**26**

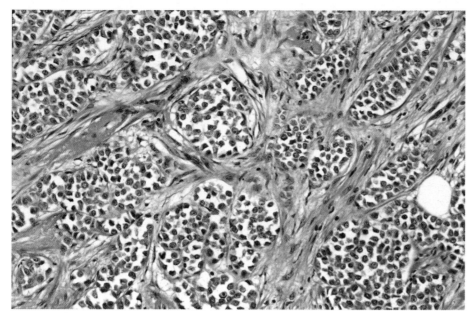

Fig. 5.**27**

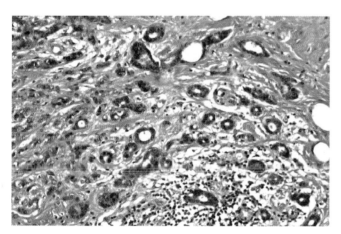

Fig. 5.**28**

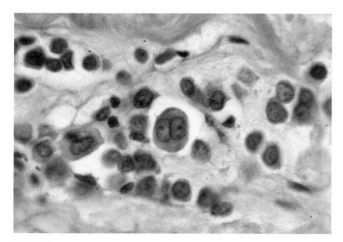

Fig. 5.**29**

More importantly, if the cells are of the lobular type, the tumors are classified as lobular carcinoma even if the cells are not growing in cell files.

1. Tumors fulfilling both criteria for lobular carcinoma are called invasive lobular carcinoma of the classic type. These tumors are composed of files of small monomorphous cells (Fig. 5.**25**).

2. A solid variant of invasive lobular carcinoma is composed of typical small monomorphous cells that grow in large solid nodules (Fig. 5.**26**).

3. An alveolar variant of invasive lobular carcinoma contains typical cells grouped in small solid nests of 10 to 20 tumor cells (Fig. 5.**27**).

4. A tubulolobular variant is composed partly of tubular structures and partly cell files of typical cells (Fig. 5.**28**). This variant has a better prognosis than the other subgroups.

5. Mixed examples of invasive lobular carcinoma containing more than one of the above-described variants are usual.

Ductal carcinomas may contain areas of classical invasive lobular carcinoma or its variants. Mixed carcinomas with clearly separated ductal and lobular component also exist. To classify a tumor as invasive lobular carcinoma, at least 90 % of the tumor should exhibit one of the patterns described above.

Invasive lobular carcinoma may form a stellate tumor body (Figs. 5.**30** and 5.**31**).

Frequently, the classic or the mixed types of invasive lobular carcinoma grow diffusely, extensively permeate the normal tissue, and form a spider's-web–like structure without a well-formed tumor body (Fig. 5.**32**). These tumors may grow to a size of several centimeters before causing any mammographic abnormality. They may be detected clinically as palpable lesions or be found by ultrasound.

The solid and mixed lobular carcinomas can form well-circumscribed, solid tumors with easily assessable size and limited extent. Even in these cases, multifocality often appears.

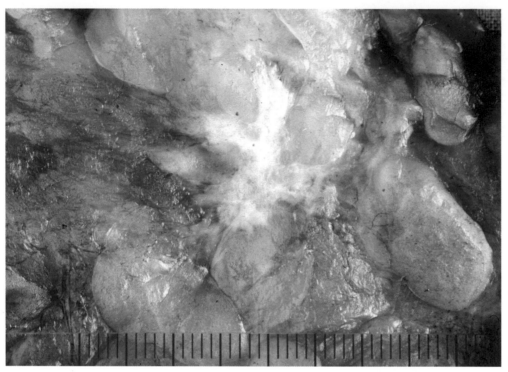

Fig. 5.**30**

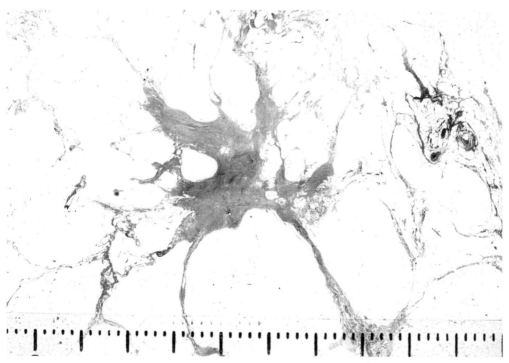

Fig. 5.**31**

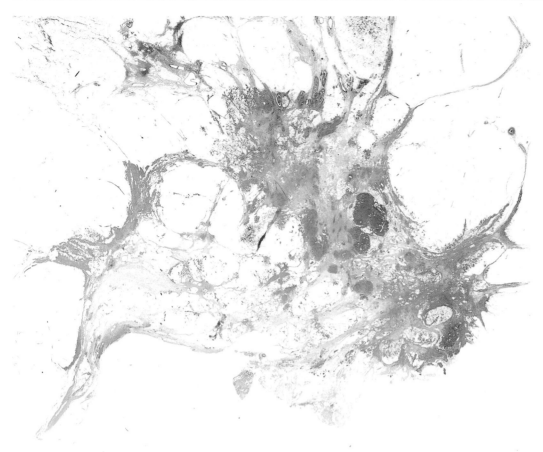

Fig. 5.32

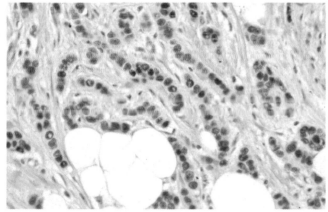

Detection of a primary and metastatic lobular carcinoma can be very difficult even on histology. Immunohisto-chemistry may be helpful in detecting the small, dispersed cells of these tumors. The cells are usually estrogen-receptor positive (Fig. 5.**33**) and react with epithelial markers (Figs. 5.**34** and 5.**35**).

Fig. 5.**33**

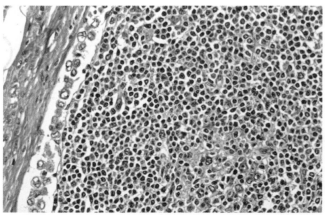

Fig. 5.**34**

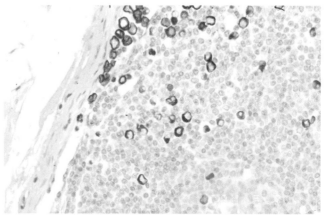

Fig. 5.**35**

Distribution of histologic types of breast cancer

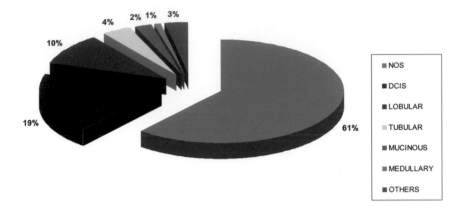

Legend:
- NOS
- DCIS
- LOBULAR
- TUBULAR
- MUCINOUS
- MEDULLARY
- OTHERS

Fig. 5.**36** (own results, 1995–98)

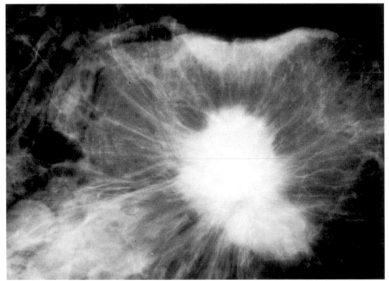

Fig. 5.**37**

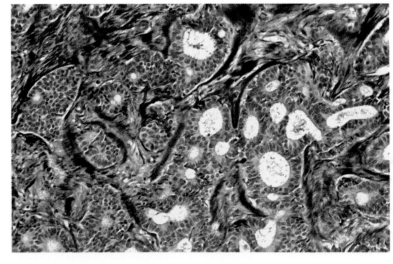

Fig. 5.**38**

This chapter is restricted to the most usual types of invasive breast carcinomas, despite the existence of many other rare tumor types. Although recognition and proper classification of these rare tumors may represent a challenge for the pathologist, the other members of the breast team are more interested in the usual morphologic prognostic parameters (size, grade, etc) even in these cases. For practical purposes, it is more important to find the similarities between the carcinoma cases than to find minor histologic differences.

As seen on the diagram above (Fig. 5.**36**), most of the invasive breast carcinomas do not fulfill the criteria of any of the breast carcinomas of special type. They belong to the category of ductal breast carcinoma "not otherwise specified" (NOS) or "no special type" (NST) (Figs. 5.**37** and 5.**38**), a large and heterogeneous group of adenocarcinomas containing more than 60% of all breast malignancies. This prognostically heterogeneous tumor group needs to be stratified by use of morphologic–prognostic factors (see Chapter 9).

Conclusions

By restrictive use of morphologic criteria, special types of mammary carcinomas can be diagnosed. Tubular and mucinous carcinomas with typical histologic patterns in at least 90% of the tumor have an excellent prognosis. Typical medullary carcinomas have better prognosis than their ductal counterparts. It is important to recognize lobular carcinomas because of the many variations of this tumor type and their tendency to be more extensive than suspected on the mammogram. Most of the invasive carcinomas, however, belong to a single large and heterogeneous group of ductal carcinoma, NOS, which has to be stratified by the use of morphologic–prognostic parameters.

References

1 Chinyama CN, Davies JD. Mammary mucinous lesions: congeners, prevalence and important pathological associations. *Histopathology.* 1996;29:533–539.
2 Toikkanen S, Pylkkänen L, Joensuu H. Invasive lobular carcinoma of the breast has better short- and long-term survival than invasive ductal carcinoma. *Br J Cancer.* 1997;76(9):1234–1240.
3 Pedersen L. Medullary carcinoma of the breast. *APMIS.* 1997;(suppl)75:105.
4 Tot T. The role of cytokeratins 20 and 7 and estrogen receptor analysis in separation of metastatic lobular carcinoma of the breast and metastatic signet ring cell carcinoma of the gastrointestinal tract. *APMIS.* 2000;108:467–472.
5 Tot T. The cytokeratin profile of medullary carcinoma of the breast. *Histopathology.* 2000;37:175–181.
6 Tabár L, et al. The Swedish Two-County Trial twenty years later. Updated mortality results and new insights from long-term follow-up. Radiol Clin North Am 38 (4):625–651:200.

Chapter 6

The Most Common Benign Breast Lesions and Their Borderline and Malignant Counterparts

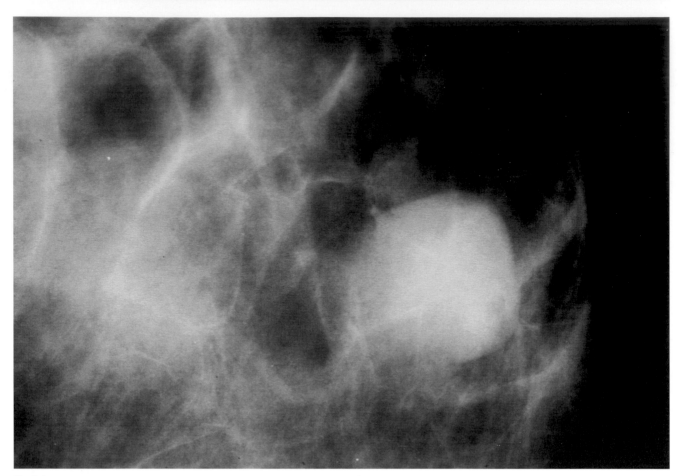

Fig. 6.**1**

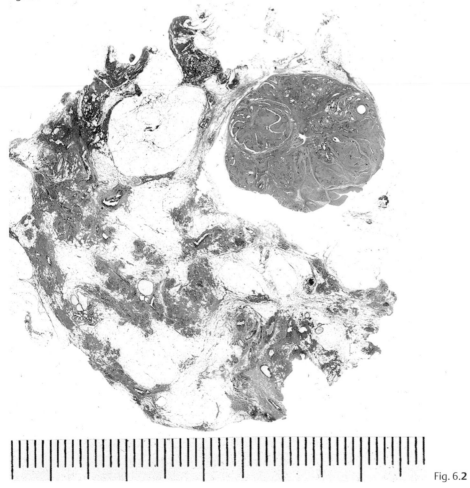

Fig. 6.**2**

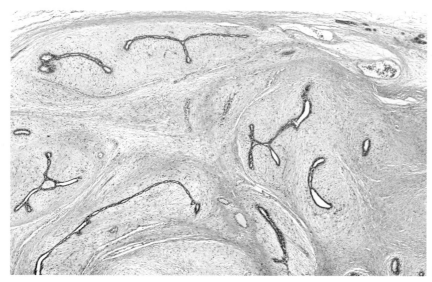

Fig. 6.**3**

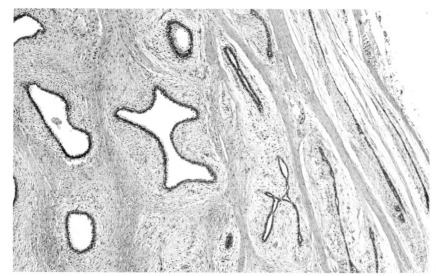

Fig. 6.**4**

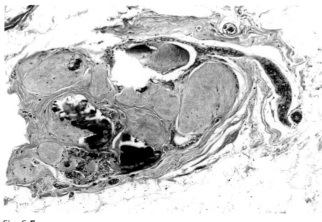

Fig. 6.**5**

Fibroadenoma (Figs. 6.**1** and 6.**2**) is a very common benign epithelial–stromal tumor mainly containing proliferated elements of the intralobular active stroma, but also featuring proliferated ducts and acini. The epithelial component is distorted in the so-called intracanalicular variant (Fig. 6.**3**) and more regular in "pericanalicular" fibroadenoma (Fig. 6.**4**). The epithelial component may exhibit hyperplastic or metaplastic changes. The stroma of the younger lesion is mucin-rich and becomes more fibrous over time. Fibroadenoma is usually a palpable lesion, but in about 10 % of the cases, it is detected on the basis of amorphous stromal microcalcifications (Fig. 6.**5**) seen on the mammogram. Fibroadenoma represents a clinically detectable phase of fibroadenomatoid change (see Chapter 1).

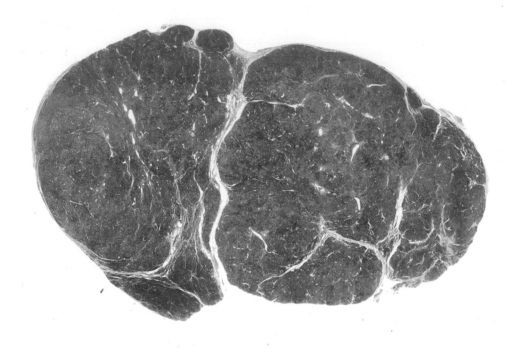

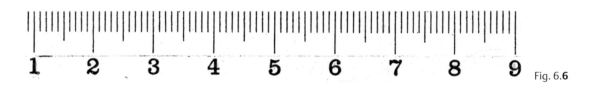

Fig. 6.**6**

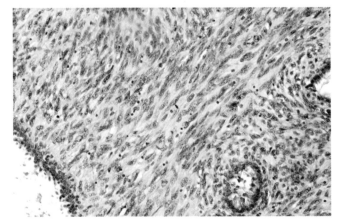

Fig. 6.**7**

The stroma in a fibroadenoma is poorly cellular and mitotically almost inactive. The "juvenile" variant of fibroadenoma is a more rapidly growing round or oval lesion that has a more cellular stroma with some mitotic figures (Fig. 6.**6**).

The term "phylloides tumor" designates a group of epithelial–stromal neoplasms with dominating stroma and leaf-like structures (Figs. 6.**7** and 6.**8**). The stroma in these lesions is more cellular and mitotically active, even in benign cases. An occurrence of more than five mitoses per ten high power fields is considered as an indicator of low malignant potential ("phylloides tumor of borderline malignancy") with a tendency to recur. Lesions with obvious stromal cellular atypia and high mitotic activity are rare and malignant. They may contain heterologeous stromal components (e.g., liposarcoma, rhabdomyosarcoma, or osteosarcoma).

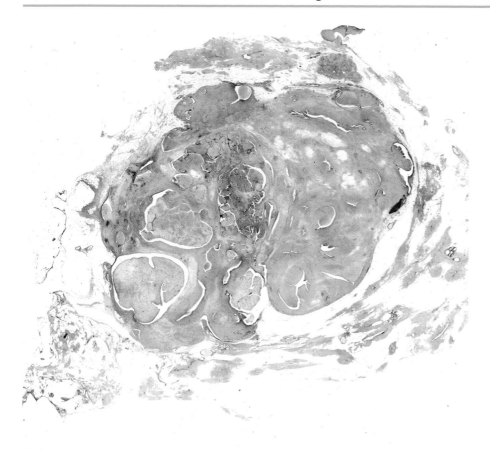

Fig. 6.8

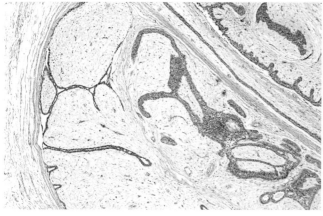

Fig. 6.9

The epithelial component of these tumors may contain foci of lobular carcinoma in situ (LCIS), ductal carcinoma in situ (DCIS) (Fig. 6.9), or invasive carcinoma.

The most important issue in this group of lesions is the potential risk of overdiagnosis. In the presence of a growing palpable mass, usually in younger women, a cellular fine-needle aspirate may lead to an erroneous preoperative diagnosis of malignancy. Core biopsy usually rules out the possibility of carcinoma and detects the rare borderline and malignant variants of these tumors.

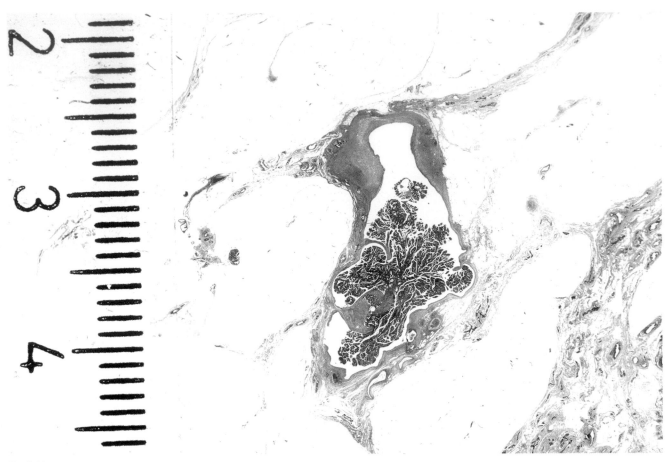

Fig. 6.**10**

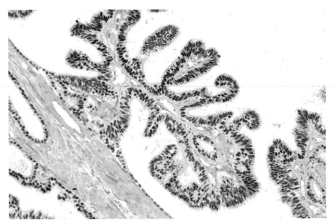

Fig. 6.**11**

One of the few lesions that originate outside the terminal ductal-lobular unit (TDLU) is a *papilloma*. It usually develops in larger ducts in the retroareolar area and often causes serous or bloody nipple discharge. Papillomas are exophytic lesions that fill the lumen of the dilated duct (Fig. 6.**10**) and contain a branching fibrous central core (Fig. 6.**11** and 6.**12**).

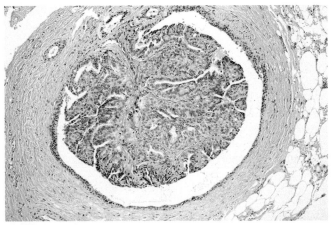

Fig. 6.**12**

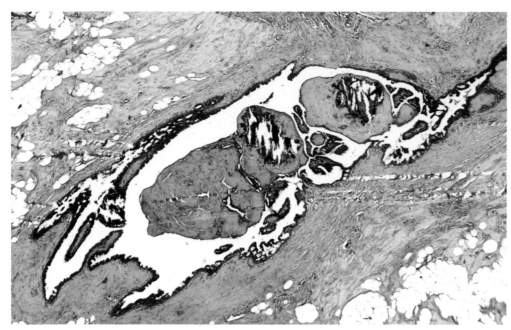

Fig. 6.**13**

The stroma of elderly papillomas may calcify (Fig. 6.**13**) and appear as a cluster of calcifications on the mammogram. However, the radiologic method of choice in detecting papillary lesions is galactography (Fig. 6.**14**).

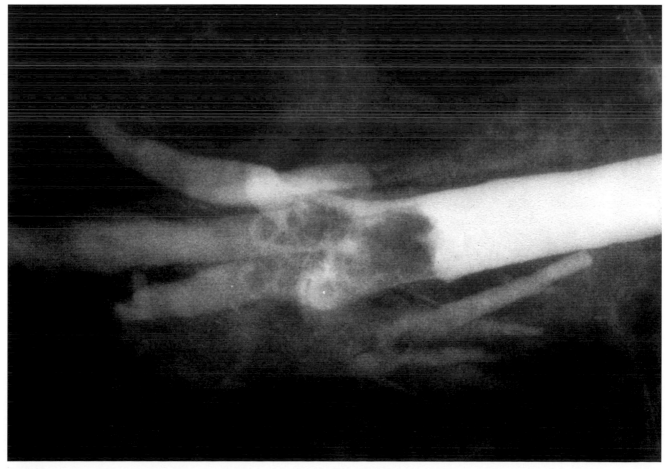

Fig. 6.**14**

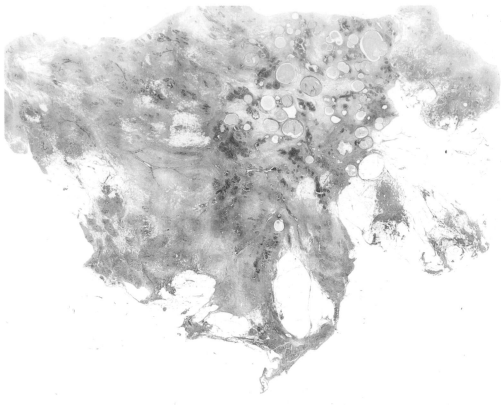

Fig. 6.**15**

Papillomas may be solitary or multiple. Sometimes in young women multiple papillomas appear in a fibrocystic area of the breast tissue. This is referred to as "juvenile papillomatosis" (Fig. 6.**15**).

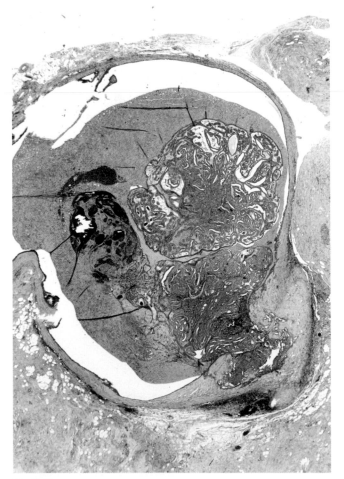

Fig. 6.**16**

The epithelial component as well as the myoepithelium in papillomas may exhibit a spectrum of metaplastic, hyperplastic and neoplastic changes resulting in benign, borderline, and malignant categories of the papillary lesions. On the benign end of the spectrum are intraductal papillomas with a single layer of epithelium and a single layer of myoepithelium, but metaplasia or hyperplasia of the epithelium and the myoepithelium frequently occurs (Fig. 6.**16**).

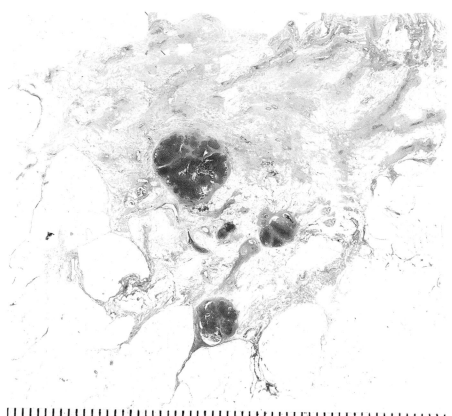

Fig. 6.**17**

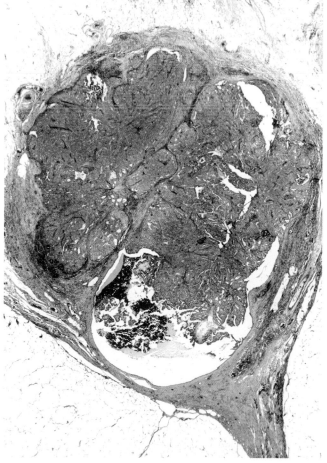

Fig. 6.**18**

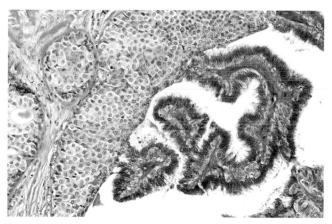

Fig. 6.**19**

The borderline category of papillary lesions is a heterogeneous group of noninfiltrating tumors with good prognosis (Figs. 6.**17**–6.**19**). They may contain foci of atypical ductal hyperplasia (ADH), DCIS, or LCIS. Terms such as "atypical papilloma" (if the malignant focus is less than 3 mm in diameter) or "malignant papilloma" (if the focus is larger) have been proposed for diagnostic use in these cases. The diagnostic criteria for hyperplasia, atypical hyperplasia, and carcinoma in situ within the papillomas are the same as those discussed in Chapter 3.

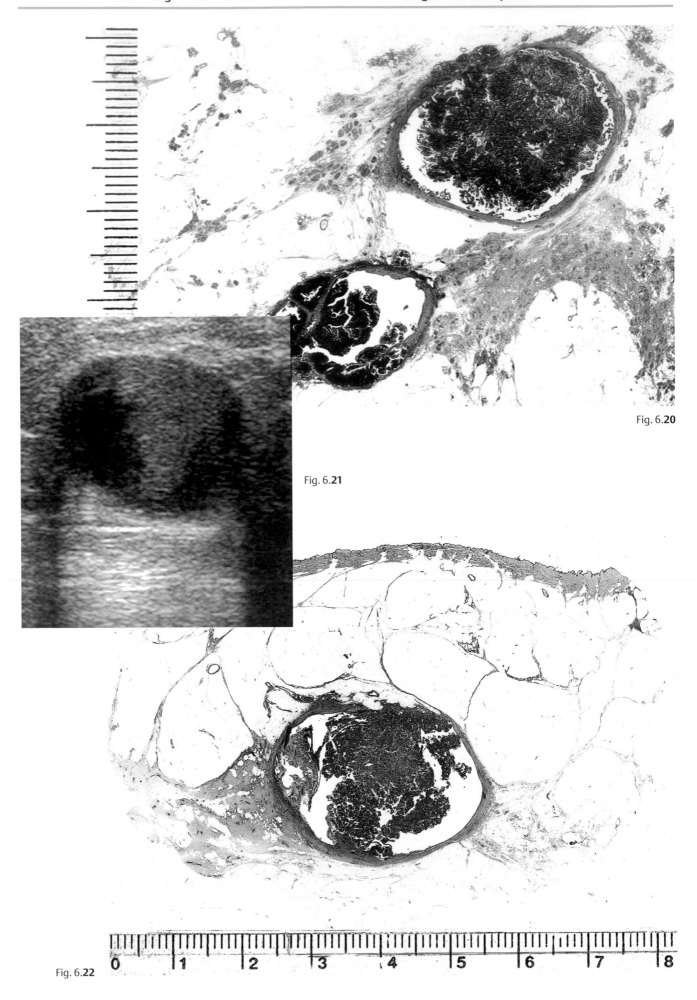

Fig. 6.**20**

Fig. 6.**21**

Fig. 6.**22**

If the duct containing a papilloma becomes cystically dilated, the lesion is designated as an intracystic papilloma (or intracystic papillary carcinoma). The intracystic papillary carcinoma contains large areas of malignant cells (usually grade I) grouped into papillary structures with a less evident fibrotic core and myoepithelium. Ordinary structures of DCIS in the TDLUs in the vicinity of the intracystic lesion, if present, represent further evidence of malignancy (Figs. 6.**20**–6.**22**).

The prognostic significance of small areas of invasion in a case of otherwise typical intracystic papillary carcinomas is unknown. If the infiltrative pattern predominates, the tumor is invasive papillary carcinoma, representing a special form of invasive breast carcinomas (Fig. 6.**23**), in which 90 % of the tumor has to exhibit a papillary pattern. The papillary pattern may be seen focally in ductal, mucinous, or mixed carcinomas. The invasive micropapillary carcinoma is another rare breast carcinoma of special type that typically consists of small papillary structures with inverse polarity of the cells (Fig. 6.**24**).

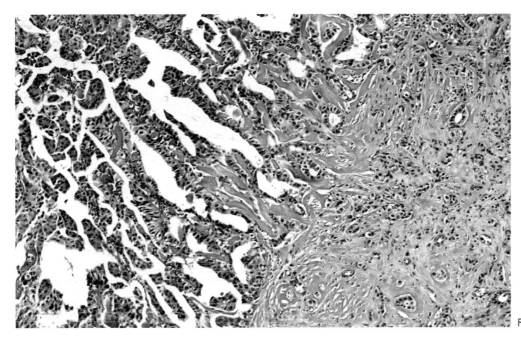

Fig. 6.**23**

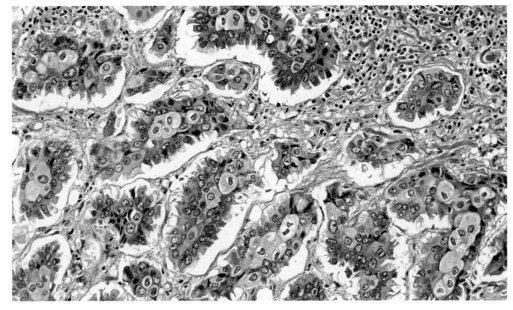

Fig. 6.**24**

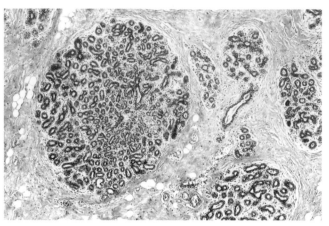

Fig. 6.**25**

While ductal hyperplasia leads to multilayering of the epithelial cells (see Chapter 3), *adenosis* represents a different form of hyperplasia resulting in increased numbers of acini per lobule, enlargement and sometimes distortion of lobules. The acini in these lesions retain the normal epithelial monolayer. There are many variations of adenosis according to the architecture and the epithelial cell characteristics. Most of them are restricted to the lobules, but some rare variants do not respect the borders of the lobules.

The most common lobulocentric variants are simple adenosis, sclerosing adenosis, and blunt duct adenosis. Simple adenosis (Fig. 6.**25**) is the prototype of these lesions: an enlarged lobule with an increased number of acini.

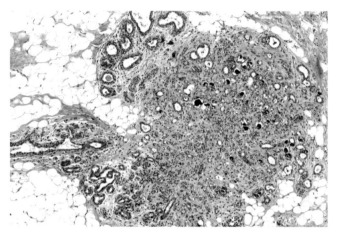

Fig. 6.**26**

In the very common sclerosing adenosis, the myoepithelium and the stromal cells also proliferate and distort the acini (Fig. 6.**26**). Sometimes on higher microscopic magnification these lesions may resemble an invasive carcinoma (Figs. 6.**27** and 6.**28**), which can be ruled out if attention is focused on lobulocentricity of these lesions.

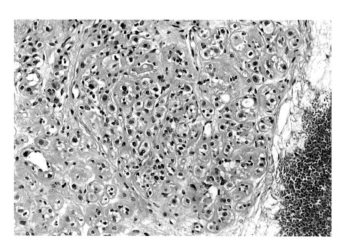

Fig. 6.**27**

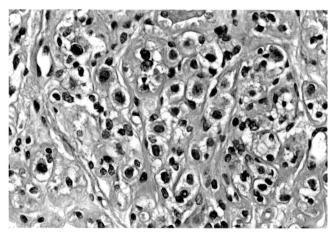

Fig. 6.**28**

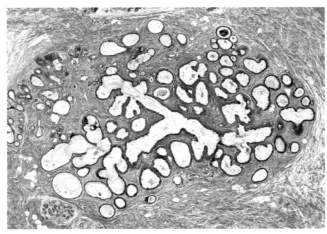

Fig. 6.**29**

The blunt duct type of adenosis has somewhat dilated acini containing high columnar epithelium (Fig. 6.**29**). In contrast to microcystic involution (Chapter 1, Figs. 1.**31** and 1.**32**), the number of acini in the lobule is not decreased.

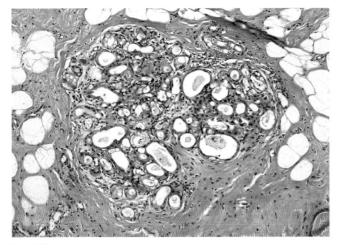

Fig. 6.**30**

The epithelium in adenosis may exhibit apocrine metaplasia and, rarely, obvious cellular atypia. These variants are designated as apocrine adenosis, atypical adenosis, or, if these cellular changes are combined, atypical apocrine adenosis (Figs. 6.**30**–6.**32**). The biologic relevance of these findings is unclear, but there is evidence to support the malignant nature of some of these lesions. Immunohistologic staining on smooth-muscle actin helps to rule out invasion in most variants of adenosis (Fig. 6.**32**).

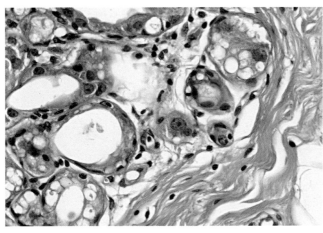

Fig. 6.**31**

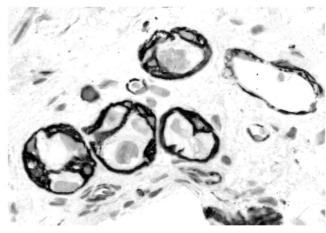

Fig. 6.**32**

Most often, adenosis represents one of the aberrations of normal development and involution (ANDI), a part of the varying picture of normal breast tissue. However, by coalescence of neighboring enlarged TDLUs, adenosis may form a palpable lesion, the so-called adenosis tumor (Fig. 6.**34**), but this is rare. More often, lobules with adenosis may contain psammoma-body–like microcalcifications (Fig. 6.**33**) which, if sufficiently numerous, can be detected on the mammogram as multifocal, lobulocentric powdery calcifications, the same type of microcalcifications as in cases of DCIS grade I (see Chapters 4 and 7).

The hallmark of the common types of adenosis is lobulocentricity. The nonlobulocentric variants (especially the so-called microglandular adenosis consisting of small uniform round acini lacking myoepithelium) always represent a differential diagnostic problem.

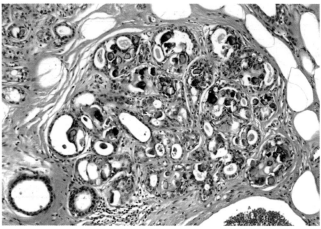

Fig. 6.**33**

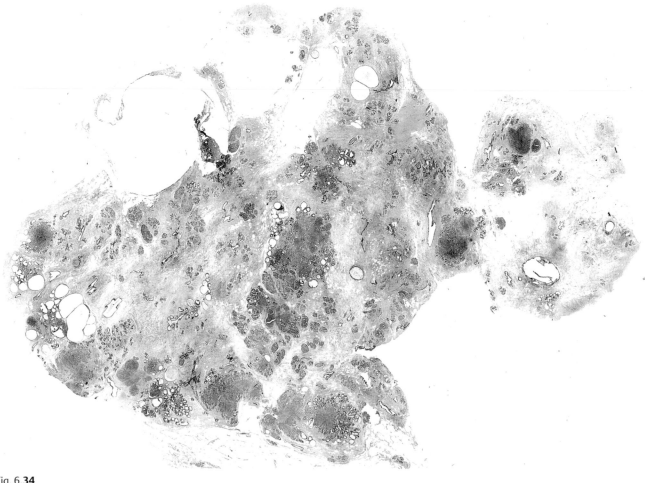

Fig. 6.**34**

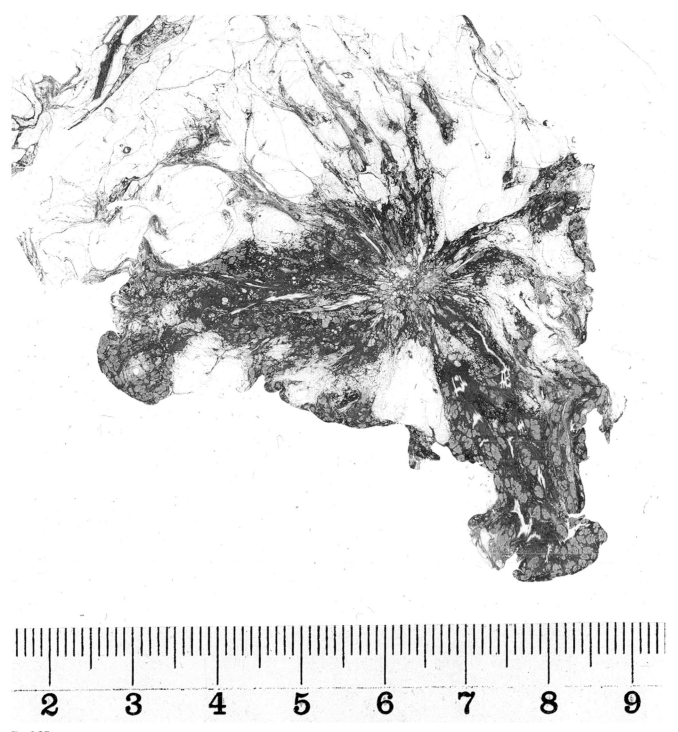

Fig. 6.**35**

Radial scars are benign lesions with a typical architecture. Centrally they contain a scleroelastic core encircled by a "corona" containing normal lobules or various ANDIs. The radial scars are most often 3 to 5-mm lesions observable only microscopically. Most of the radiologically detected lesions are 15 to 20-mm, nonpalpable, stellate lesions (Figs. 6.**35**–6.**39**). Sometimes even larger radial scars may develop, which are synonymously called "complex sclerosing lesions."

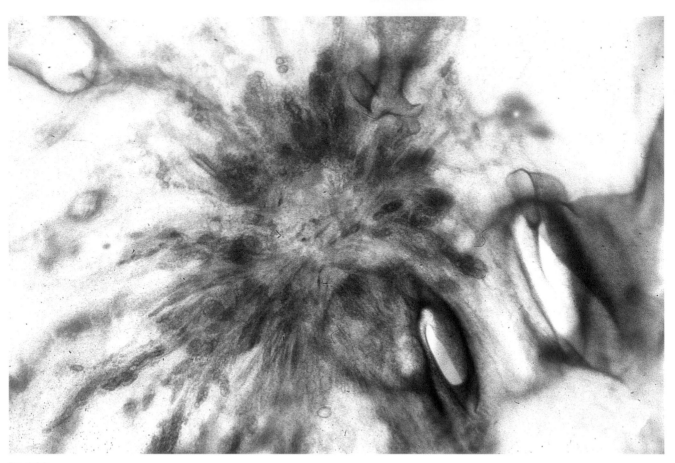

Fig. 6.**36**

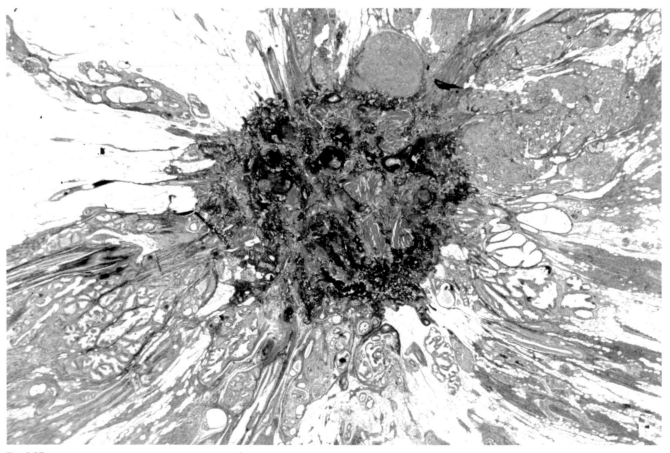

Fig. 6.**37**

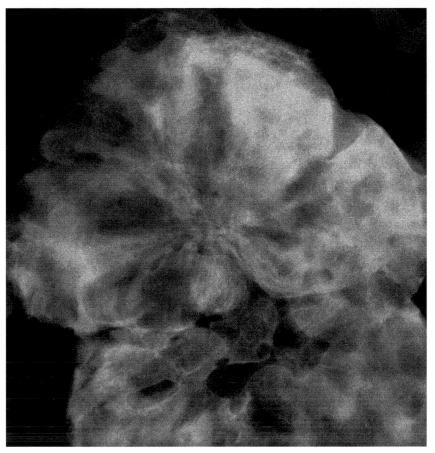

Fig. 6.**38**

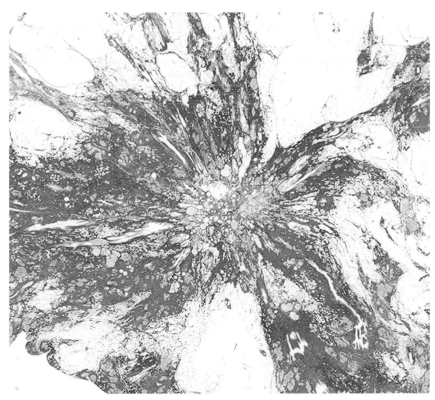

Fig. 6.**39**

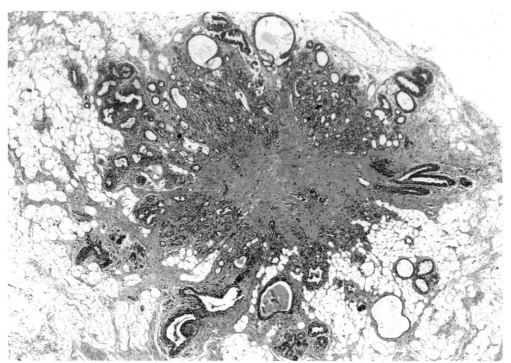

Fig. 6.**40**

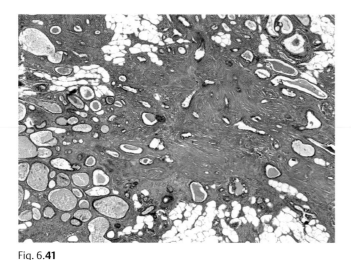

Fig. 6.**41**

In a considerable proportion of cases, the corona of the radial scars may contain a monotonous population of low-grade cancer cells filling the lobules in a form of atypical lobular hyperplasia (ALH), LCIS, ADH, or DCIS grade I. Because these lesions represent the "borderline area" of malignancy and are usually focal or multifocal, a small sample of the tissue from the corona (e.g., a core biopsy) may not be representative.

Accumulation of elastic fibers in the middle of the lesion usually distorts the pre-existing ducts, which may imitate invasion. Because these pseudoinvasive glands lack cellular atypia, the differential diagnostic options include tubular carcinoma or ductal carcinoma "not otherwise specified" (NOS) grade I. The glands in the scleroelastic core of radial scars usually retain the myoepithelial cell layer and do not invade the surrounding fatty tissue (Figs. 6.**40** and 6.**41**).

Because they are nonpalpable, radial scars are preoperatively detected by mammography. These lesions are typically stellate with a central radiolucent area (the so-called black star, Fig. 6.**42**) and differ in their radiologic appearance from invasive carcinomas having a central radiopaque and usually palpable tumor body (the so-called white star, Fig. 6.**43**).

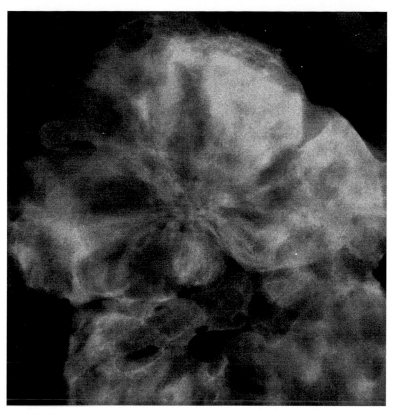

Fig. 6.**42**

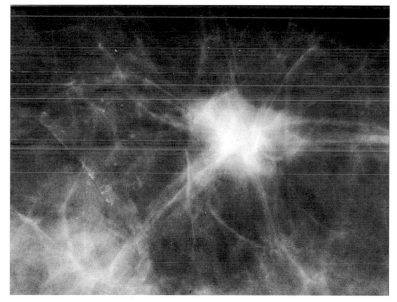

Fig. 6.**43**

Conclusions

In addition to fibrocystic change (see Chapter 1), fibroadenomas, papillomas, different types of adenosis, and radial scars are the most commonly seen benign breast lesions. A detailed histologic work-up of these lesions is needed because they may contain foci of malignant cells and because they have rare malignant variants. Some of these lesions have to be included in the differential diagnosis of certain forms of invasive and in situ carcinomas, and some are regarded as a special type of DCIS.

References

1 Page DL, et al. Subsequent breast carcinoma risk after biopsy with atypia in a breast papilloma. *Cancer.* 1996;78:258–266.
2 Seidman JD, Ashton M, Lefkowitz M. Atypical apocrine adenosis of the breast. *Cancer.* 1996;77:2529–2537.
3 Lopez-Ferrer P, et al. Fine needle aspiration cytology of the breast fibroadenoma. A cytohistologic correlation study of 405 cases. *Acta Cytol.* 1999;43:579–586.
4 Tabár L, Dean PB, Tot T. Teaching atlas of mammography. 3rd ed. Stuttgart, New York: Georg Thieme Verlag: 2001.

Chapter 7

Fine-needle Aspiration or Core Biopsy: A Preoperative Diagnostic Algorithm

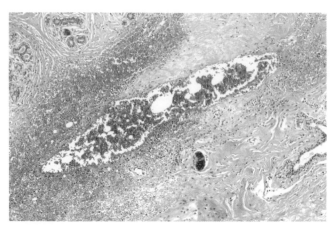

Fig. 7.**1**

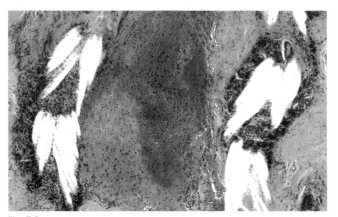

Fig. 7.**2**

Any procedure involving use of a needle causes mechanical damage to the targeted tissue. The same is true in cases of fine-needle aspiration or core biopsy of the breast. Necrosis, needle tracks containing blood (Fig. 7.**1**), inflammatory cells, or cholesterol crystals (Fig. 7.**2**) are the most common findings.

Sometimes an inflammatory pseudotumor forms around the damage (Fig. 7.**3**), with hemosiderin-containing macrophages surrounding the needle tracks (Fig. 7.**4**).

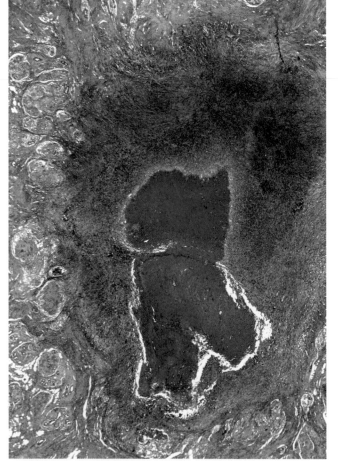

Fig. 7.**3**

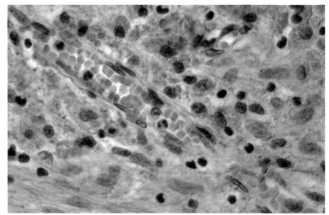

Fig. 7.**4**

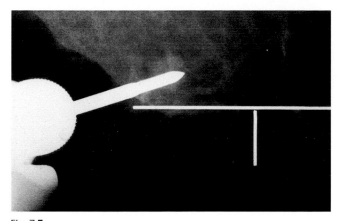

Fig. 7.**5**

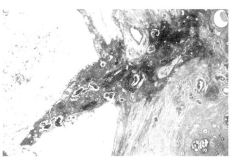

Fig. 7.**7**

Epithelial displacement may make it difficult for the pathologist to determine the extent of invasion (Figs. 7.**6** and 7.**7**).

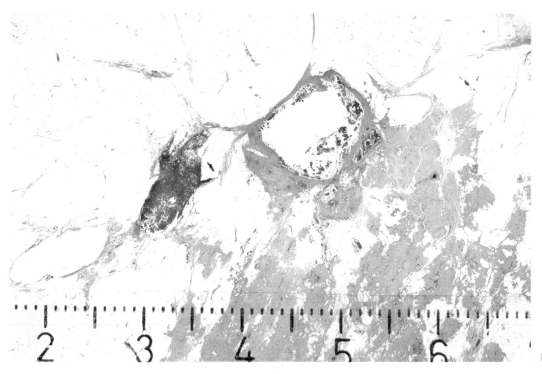

Fig. 7.**6**

There is insufficient evidence to determine whether or not a needling procedure can initiate metastatic tumor spread, but this possibility cannot be ruled out. Because of this uncertainty, we recommend a restrictive approach when using these procedures.

The aim of the diagnostic needling procedure is to obtain the minimum representative tissue needed for a definite preoperative diagnosis, while at the same time causing the least harm to the patient (compare Figs. 7.**8** and 7.**9**).

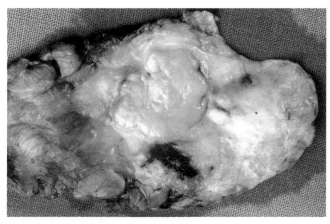

Fig. 7.**8**

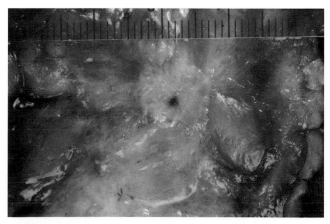

Fig. 7.**9**

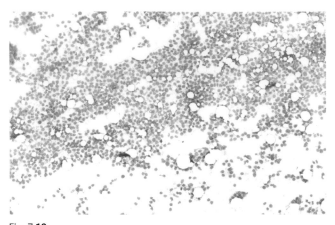

Fig. 7.**10**

Fig. 7.**11**

Fine-needle aspiration biopsy (FNAB) is a simple, quick, and very useful method for the preoperative diagnosis of breast lesions. In experienced hands, when used in conjunction with clinical and radiologic findings, FNAB has high sensitivity, specificity, and accuracy.

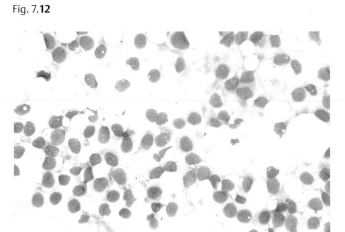

Fig. 7.**12**

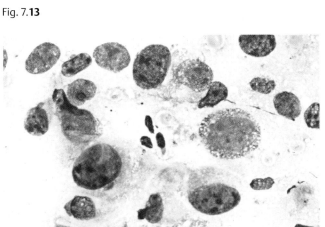

Fig. 7.**13**

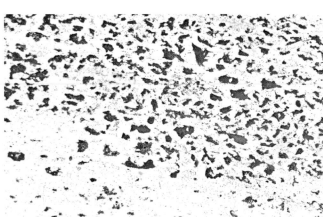

Fig. 7.**14**

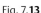

Fig. 7.**15**

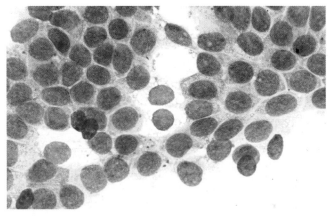

Fig. 7.**16**

Fig. 7.**17**

The most useful cytologic diagnostic criteria of malignancy are:

– *high cellularity* (compare Figs. 7.**10** and 7.**11**)

– *absence of myoepithelial cells* (seen best in benign lesions as small, oval, bare nuclei, single or in pairs, in the background of the smear [Fig. 7.**12**])

– *loss of cohesiveness* of the epithelial cells (compare Figs. 7.**13** and 7.**14**), and

– *cellular atypia* (compare Figs. 7.**15** and 7.**16**).

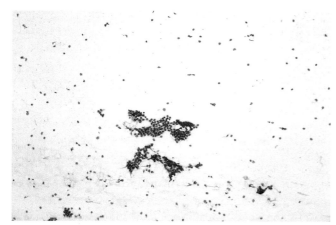

Fig. 7.**18**

The goals of FNAB are not to rule out, but to verify a malignancy, if possible, and to categorize the cytologic picture rather than to type and grade the lesions. FNAB categorizes the cytologic picture as follows:

II: unsatisfactory sample (Fig. 7.**17**)

III: benign, no cytologic signs of malignancy (Fig. 7.**18**)

IV: suspicious for malignancy (Fig. 7.**19**), or

V: malignant (Fig. 7.**20**).

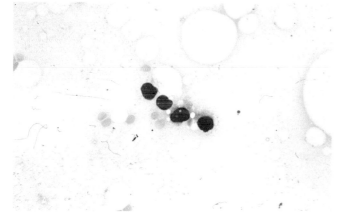

Fig. 7.**19**

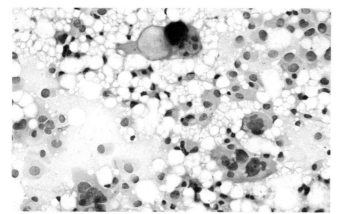

Fig. 7.**20**

Category I is reserved for cases without preoperative FNAB (see Fig. 7.**23**).

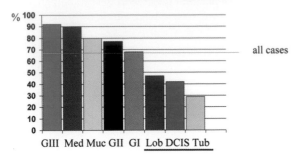

Diagnostic accuracy of FNAB in 240 breast cancers

Fig. 7.**21**

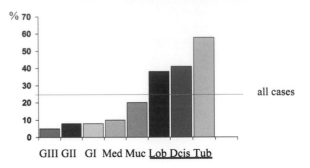

FNAB negatives (II+III) 37/240 breast cancer cases

Fig. 7.**22**

Quality assurance program 96

Histologic outcome

	I	II	III	IV	V
I					
II					
III					
IV					
V					

(FNAB)

I   not done
II unsatisfactory
III benign
IV suspicious
V   malignant

Fig. 7.**23**

Figures 7.**21** and 7.**22** show our data on the accuracy of FNAB according to tumor grade and type. While grade III carcinomas and medullary and mucinous carcinomas are easy to sample and interpret, the opposite is true for invasive lobular carcinomas, tubular carcinomas, and ductal carcinoma in situ (DCIS). The cytologist has to continuously follow up the results of preoperative FNAB comparing them to the postoperative histologic outcome. A simple method of comparison uses the table shown in Figure 7.**23**. On the basis of these data, statistical parameters such as sensitivity, specificity, accuracy, and false-negative and false-positive rates can be calculated. An unsatisfactory rate less than 20%, absolute sensitivity over 60%, and complete sensitivity (malignant + suspicious FNABs/malignant outcome) over 80% are the suggested minimum standards. Most importantly, the false-positive rate must be as near to zero as possible.

Average accuracy FNAB:CORE

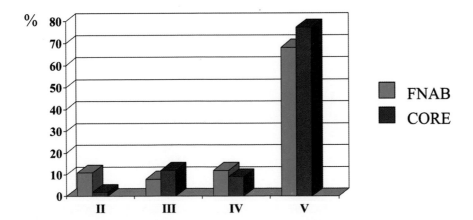

Fig. 7.**24**

Core-needle biopsy allows definitive preoperative histo-logic diagnoses in most of the representative sample cases (Figs. 7.25 and 7.26). This procedure has a slightly higher average accuracy compared to FNAB (Fig. 7.24). We found this procedure to be particularly useful in cases of lobular invasive carcinoma, tubular carcinoma, and DCIS (Fig. 7.5).

Another advantage of core-needle biopsy is that benign conditions, especially fibroadenoma, can be easily diag-nosed (see Chapter 6).

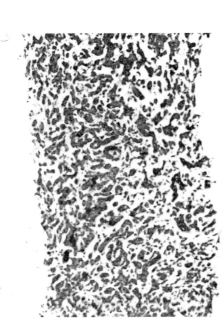

Fig 7.25

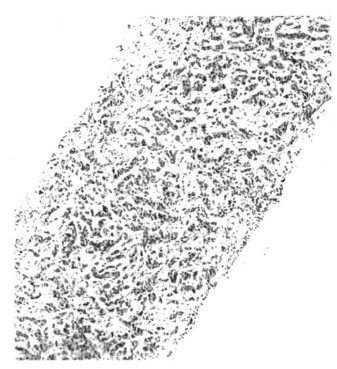

Fig. 7.26

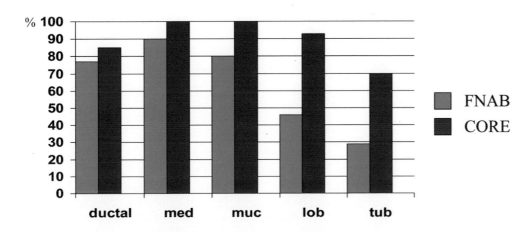

Fig. 7.27

Preoperative Diagnostic Algorithm

Most of the operated breast lesions in a properly functioning breast center will be malignant. About 75% of the lesions referred to surgical intervention, benign and malignant combined, will be circular or stellate masses on the mammogram with or without associated microcalcifications. Nearly 25% of the operated lesions will be microcalcifications on the mammogram without an associated tumor mass. Approximately 3% of the cases will be operated on after galactography.

A *Round/oval-shaped densities* on the mammogram (Fig. 7.**28**).

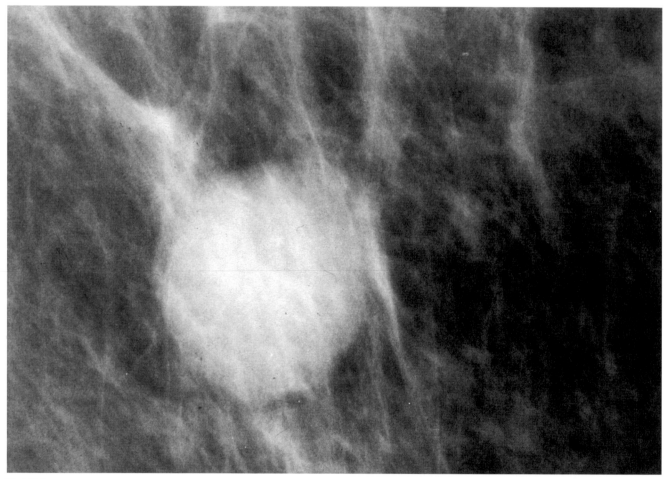

Fig. 7.**28**

Only about 60% of the operated circular or oval lesions will be malignant. The benign portion consists mostly of fibroadenoma, fibrocystic change and papilloma. Most of the cysts should be treated by aspiration, and they are not included in the percentage of the benign operated circular lesions.

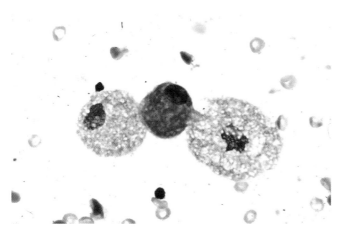

Fig. 7.**29**

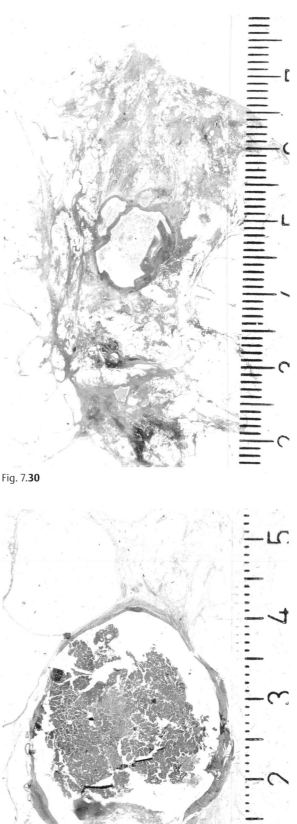

A1 Cystic by ultrasound examination.

A1a When ultrasound examination shows no intracystic growth, cyst aspiration depends on clinical setting and patient concerns. Cytologic examination of the fluid removed from a simple cyst is not necessary. The cytologic image otherwise shows low cellularity, foam cells and apocrine cells (Figs. 7.**29** and 7.**30**).

A1b When ultrasound examination shows intracystic growth, fine-needle aspiration and/or core biopsy are unreliable methods and may cause pseudoinvasion. Open surgical biopsy and histologic examination of the lesion and the surrounding tissue is necessary to arrive at definite diagnosis (see Chapter 6). Intracystic papillary tumor may be suspected on the base of large papillary cellgroups in the aspirated fluid (Figs. 7.**31** and 7.**32**).

Fig. 7.**30**

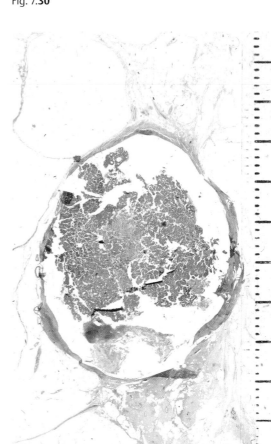

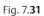

Fig. 7.**31**

Fig. 7.**32**

A2   Round/oval radiopaque densities on the mammogram, *solid* on ultrasound.

A2a Clinically and/or mammographically *malignant = perform fine-needle aspiration.*
Cytologically malignant = definite diagnosis.
Cytologically suspicious on malignancy = perform core biopsy.
Cytologically benign = perform core biopsy.
Inadequate material aspirated = repeat the aspiration.

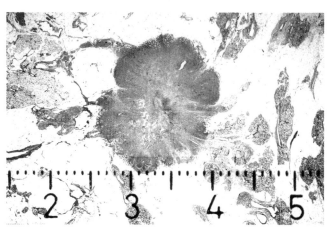

Fig. 7.**33**

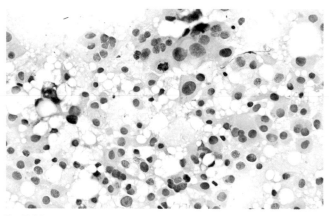

Fig. 7.**34**

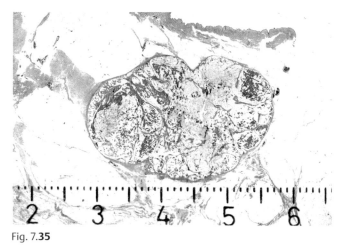

Fig. 7.**35**

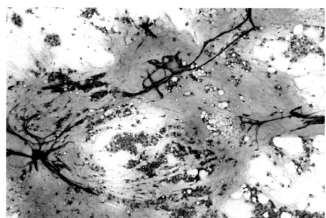

Fig. 7.**36**

A2b Clinically and mammographically *benign = perform core biopsy.*

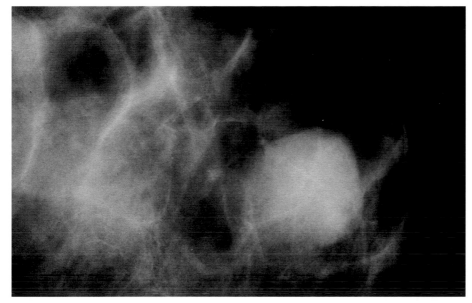

Fig. 7.**37**

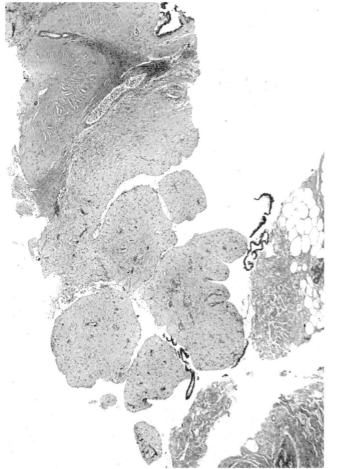

Fig. 7.**38**

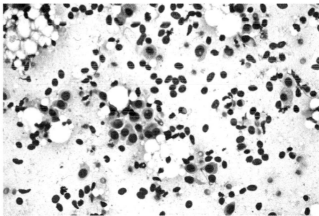

Fig. 7.**39**

Comment

The malignant round or oval lesions will most often be invasive ductal not otherwise specified (NOS) carcinomas grade II or III (Figs. 7.**33** and 7.**34**), medullary or mucinous carcinomas. They can be diagnosed easily by fine-needle aspiration because of their cellularity, obvious cellular atypia, and, in the case of mucinous carcinoma, from the presence of mucin (Figs. 7.**35** and 7.**36**). The most commonly encountered benign circular solid lesion is a fibroadenoma (Fig. 7.**37**). It is easily diagnosed on core biopsy (Fig. 7.**38**) but cytology often provides a cellular picture with moderate atypia; this is the most common source of a false-positive FNAB diagnosis (Fig. 7.**39**).

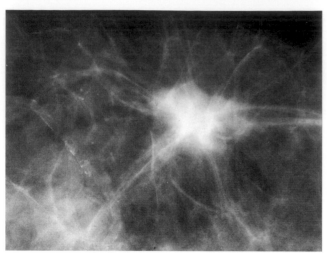

Fig. 7.**40**

B   *Stellate lesions* on the mammogram.
The stellate lesions will be malignant in over 90% of the cases, and the rest will mostly be cases of radial scars.

B1   *"A white star"* (Fig. 7.**40**) = *perform fine-needle aspiration.*
Cytologically malignant = definite diagnosis. Core biopsy adds information about the invasive nature, histologic grade and type of the lesion.
Cytologically suspicious on malignancy = perform core biopsy.
Cytologically benign = perform core biopsy.
Inadequate material aspirated = perform core biopsy.

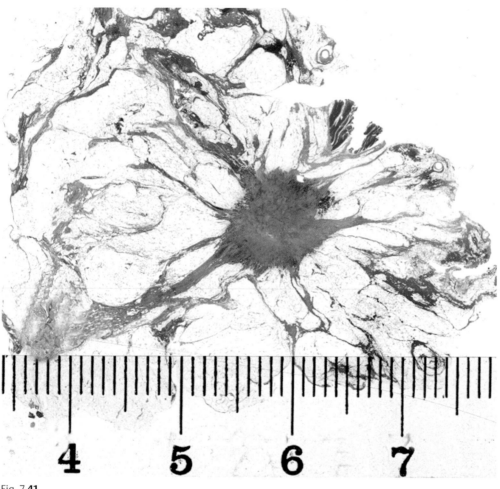

Fig. 7.**41**

Comment

"White stars" on the mammogram are nearly always malignant, most often ductal NOS carcinomas grades I (Fig. 7.**41**) and II, tubular or lobular carcinomas. Stromal desmoplasia may make it difficult to obtain representative cytologic material by fine-needle aspiration. Satisfactory cellularity cannot be expected even if the aspiration is repeated. The rare posttraumatic or postoperative stellate scar tissue (Fig. 7.**44**) may cause differential diagnostic difficulties.

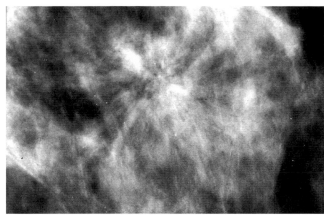

Fig. 7.**42**

B2 *"Black star"* (Fig. 7.**42**) = *perform an open surgical biopsy.*

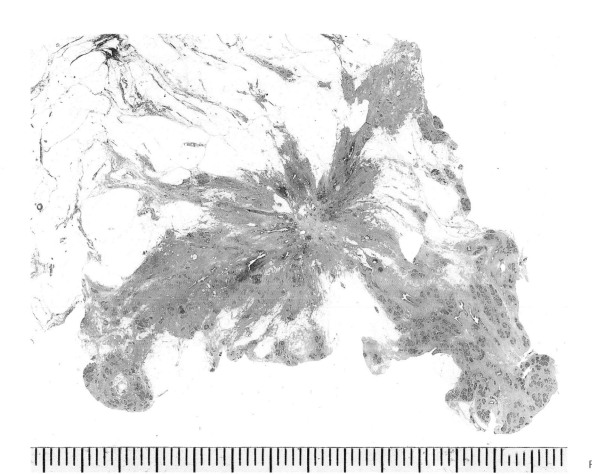

Fig. 7.**43**

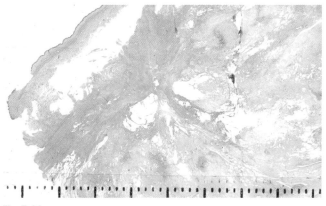

Fig. 7.**44**

Comment

The black stars on the mammogram will be radial scars (Fig. 7.**43**), which may contain foci of ductal hyperplasia, atypical ductal hyperplasia (ADH), atypical lobular hyperplasia (ALH), lobular carcinoma in situ (LCIS), or DCIS grade I in the "crown." In the fibroelastic center, pseudoinfiltrative tubular structures may be present, simulating tubular cancer (see Chapter 6). Cytology is not the method of choice for making the diagnosis of these low-grade lesions. Even core biopsy may provide insufficient material for the differential diagnosis of the above-mentioned lesions. The method of choice is large-section histology of the entire lesion.

C   *Microcalcifications* on the mammogram.

C1   *"Casting type"* (Fig. 7.**45**) (96% probability of malignancy) = perform fine-needle aspiration or core biopsy.

C2   *"Broken-needle type"* (Fig. 7.**46**) (60% probability of malignancy) = perform larger bore-needle biopsy.

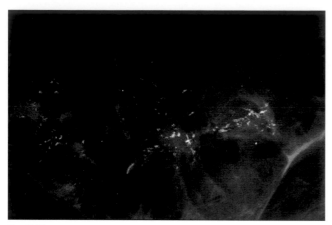

Fig. 7.**45**

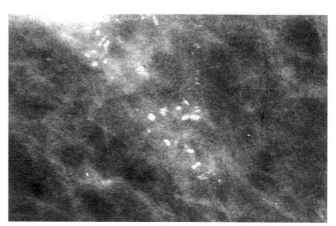

Fig. 7.**46**

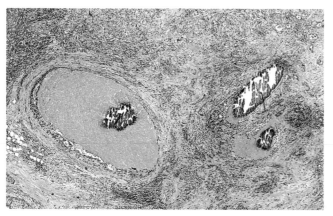

Fig. 7.**47**

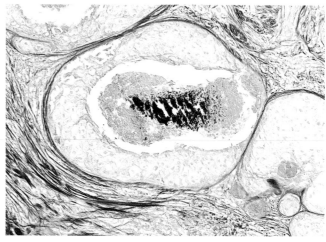

Fig. 7.**48**

Comment

These calcifications almost always represent DCIS grade III (or II) with or without invasion (Fig. 7.**47**). A definite preoperative morphologic diagnosis of malignancy can often be made with cytology because the tumor cells are highly atypical. If it is necessary to prove the presence of invasion preoperatively, core biopsy is required, but its relatively low sensitivity for small foci of invasion must be kept in mind. Surgical intervention is always necessary.

Comment

These microcalcifications often indicate DCIS grade II, engaging an enlarged lobule (Fig. 7.**48**). Differential diagnosis include papillomas, fibroadenomas, and cases of fibrocystic change (see also comment under **C1** about invasion and Chapter 4).

C3 *"Powdery"* microcalcifications (Fig. 7.**49**) (45% probability of malignancy) = perform wide open surgical biopsy.

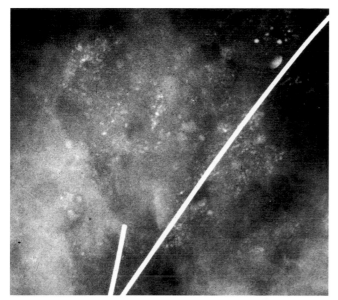

Fig. 7.**49**

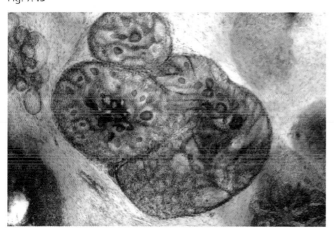

Fig. 7.**50**

Conclusions

This preoperative diagnostic algorithm represents a synthesis of our knowledge about the clinical, mammographic, and histologic characteristics of breast diseases. It also represents a rational method for using preoperative diagnostic procedures such as fine-needle aspiration biopsy, core biopsy, and surgical excisional biopsy. The preoperative diagnostic procedure has to be as harmless as possible for the patient and cause as few as possible changes to the tumor. A gentle fine-needle aspiration can give adequate diagnostic material to prove the clinical and mammographic diagnosis of malignancy. Fibroadenomas and papillomas may yield cellular and atypical aspirates, which in turn may lead to a false-positive cytologic diagnosis. Core biopsy has a better ability to prove the benign nature of the lesions. On the other hand, ruling out malignancy is sometimes, especially in low-grade lesions, impossible by FNAB or core biopsy. In these cases, wide surgical excision is indicated. Most importantly, the pathologist must correlate his or her findings with radiologic findings and understand the clinical relevance of all the details in the pathologic report.

Comment

This mammographic picture indicates the presence of a large number of psammoma body-like microcalcifications in the lumina of the altered terminal ductal-lobular units (TDLUs). This can usually be observed in different types of adenosis, mainly sclerosing adenosis, apocrine metaplasia, but even in DCIS grade I (Fig. 7.**50**, thick-section image). Fine-needle aspiration is inadequate for assessing this grade of DCIS because the cells are highly differentiated. The microcalcifications may be localized in benign structures adjacent to the DCIS and not in the DCIS itself, so that a mammographically directed core biopsy may give a false-negative result.

References

1 Willis SL, Ramzy I. Analysis of false results in a series of 835 fine needle aspirates of breast lesions. *Acta Cytol.* 1999;39:858–864.
2 Tot T, Tabár L, Gere M. The role of core needle biopsy of breast lesions when fine needle aspiration biopsy is inconclusive [summary]. *Acta Cytol.* 1999;43(4).
3 Tabár L, et al. A new era in the diagnosis of breast cancer. *Surg Oncol Clin North Am.* 2000;9(2):233–277.

Chapter 8

The Postoperative
Work-up

To determine the real extent, size, and distribution of the lesions in the excised breast tissue, the histologic findings need to be directly correlated with the clinical, mammographic, and macroscopic findings. To accomplish this correlation, the pathologist should prepare and examine sections of tissue that are as large and as continuous as possible. To this end, the technique of large histologic sections is unquestionably superior to the traditional small-block technique.

The production of a two-dimensional large-section image needs to be carefully planned. The method of the cut up of the specimen differs according to the type of the operation (mastectomy or segmentectomy/quadrantectomy) and lesion (microcalcifications, solitary or multiple tumors).

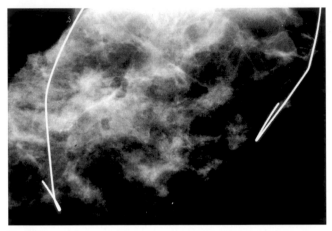

Fig. 8.**1**

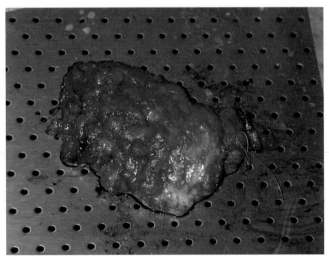

Fig. 8.**2**

The specimen is received in a fresh state after specimen radiography is performed to confirm the presence of the preoperatively diagnosed radiologic abnormality within it. The specimen radiogram (Fig. 8.**1**) assists the pathologist in planning the cut-up to include a transsection of the entire abnormality in a single large section. Thorough macroscopic examination of the specimen is also important. The size of the specimen should be measured in three dimensions, and the number and type of the marking sutures (Fig. 8.**3**) and the number and position of the guide wires should be recorded. Because the specimen consists of soft breast tissue atop a firm base (radiograph film, table), it usually takes the form of a relatively flat piece of tissue (Figs. 8.**2** and 8.**3**). The larger tumors are firmer and are usually easily located by inspection and palpation. The smaller tumors are not directly seen on macroscopic examination of the unsliced specimen, but are often palpable and are usually easily seen on the specimen radiograph. If the specimen contains only radiologically detected microcalcifications or a small nonpalpable tumor, finding the appropriate plane for slicing is totally dependent upon careful mammographic guidance. In the latter situation, it is best to slice the specimen horizontally (parallel with the table) in the plane of the specimen radiograph (Figs. 8.**4** and 8.**5**). This is recommended even in the presence of a solitary well-defined tumor mass. Multiple tumors are more difficult to demonstrate in a single large section. In these cases, the plane for the slicing should be chosen on the basis of palpation of the entire specimen and on evaluation of the specimen radiograph.

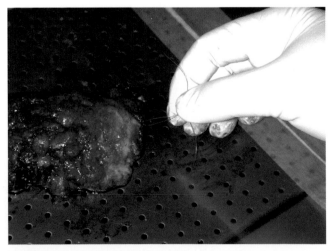

Fig. 8.**3**

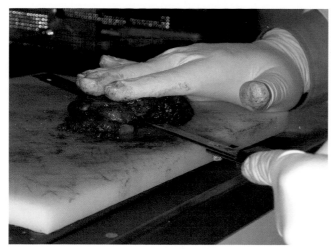

Fig. 8.**4**

For adequate slicing of a fresh breast specimen, a special knife with a very sharp disposable blade is needed. The blade must be changed after every two or three breast specimens are cut, more often when very hard or calcified tissue is encountered. It is more dangerous for the pathologist to use a dull blade than to use a very sharp one. Inexperienced pathologists are advised to use a translucent plastic plate to push the specimen against the table instead of holding it directly with their hand (Fig. 8.**6**).

The slices should be 3 to 4-mm thick (Figs. 8.**7** and 8.**8**). A considerable variation in thickness within the same slice or among slices can markedly reduce the technical quality of the specimen mammograms and histologic sections. The slices need to be thoroughly examined macroscopically. The well-formed tumor masses should be described and measured in millimeters. The relation of the tumors to the resection margins must be described in terms of the minimum number of millimeters of tumor-free margins. A lengthy macroscopic description is unnecessary because the cut surface of the entire specimen is demonstrated on the large histologic sections.

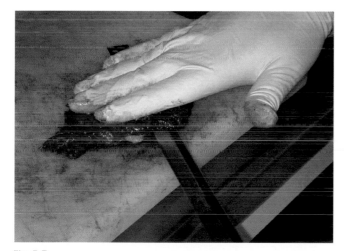

Fig. 8.**5**

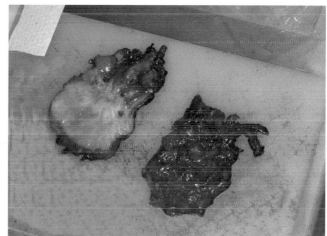

Fig. 8.**7**

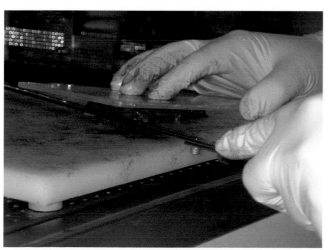

Fig. 8.**6**

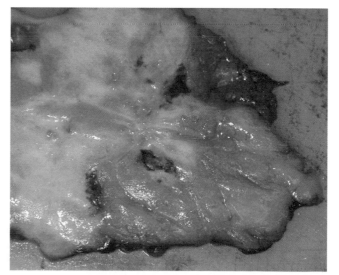

Fig. 8.**8**

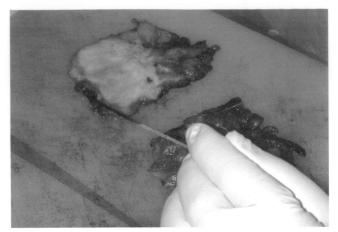

Fig. 8.**9**

Inking of the surface of the specimen is not necessary with this technique, but colored inks should be used to mark the position of the marking sutures (Fig. 8.**9**).

The 3 to 4-mm slices then undergo repeat specimen radiography. The radiographic examination of the slices (Fig. 8.**10**) is always a useful procedure and is absolutely necessary in cases with mammographically detected microcalcifications, those with multifocal tumors, and those with nonpalpable lesions. The radiologist compares the mammographic findings and the findings on specimen radiography with the radiologic images of the macroslices, and then marks the slices that have radiologic abnormalities. The pathologist must correlate the macroscopic findings in the marked slices with the radiologic abnormalities. The most representative slices are selected for imbedding and processing: the slices with the largest tumor diameter, those containing the largest number of tumor foci in the cases with multifocal tumors, those containing macroscopically and/or radiologically discernible nonmalignant lesions, and those containing microcalcifications. It is worth mentioning that pathologists are fully responsible for tissue sampling, even with radiologic assistance. Therefore, they are encouraged to sample all suspicious macroscopic abnormalities, even those that have not been marked by the radiologist.

The recommended average number of selected slices per case is two to four. At this step, small tissue blocks may be taken for immunohistology, image analysis, flow cytometry, and molecular biologic examinations, but the most representative slices must be left intact. Because the reliability of the histologic diagnosis of mammographically detected and macroscopically poorly defined lesions depends upon mammographic–pathologic correlation, one adequate large section is more important than the additional examinations. In these cases, especially if the lesion is smaller than 10 mm in the largest dimension, sampling of the tumor tissue for special examinations or taking intraoperative frozen sections is contraindicated.

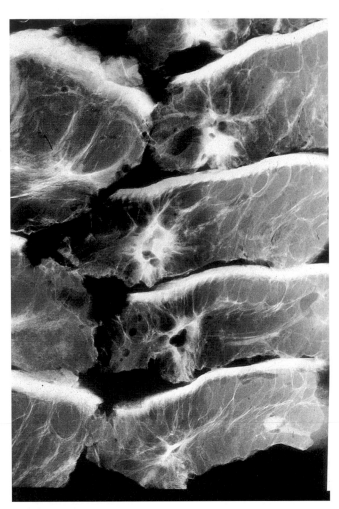

Fig. 8.**10**

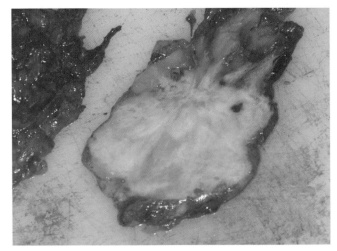

Fig. 8.**11**

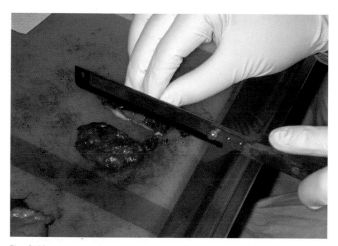

Fig. 8.**12**

Large histologic sections provide an ideal tool for assessing the circumferential resection margins. The superficial and the deep resection margins are not directly demonstrated because the specimen is sectioned horizontally. Absence of radiologic and macroscopic abnormalities in the first and the last horizontally taken slice provides indirect proof that the margins are free of tumor along both these surfaces. Should one or both of these slices contain a tumor or other abnormality, it is necessary to complete the sampling of the tissue by small tissue blocks that demonstrate the margins over and under the tumor (Fig. 8.**12**).

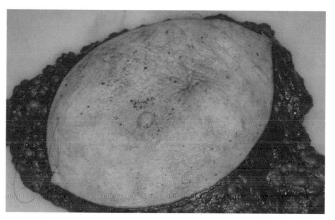

Fig. 8.**13**

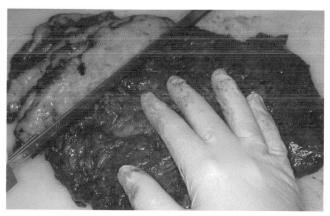

Fig. 8.**14**

Slicing the mastectomy specimen (Fig. 8.**13**) for large-section histology is a different procedure for two practical reasons: the cut surface of the specimen is usually much larger than the dimensions of the routinely used large-section glasses and, more importantly, the posterior resection margin (and not the circumferential as in segmentectomy) is the only important one in the case of mastectomy. Therefore, the large section must demonstrate the posterior surgical margin. The specimen is sliced sagitally (in a plane perpendicular to the resection margin of the mastectomy specimen) (Figs. 8.**14** and 8.**15**). Parallel slices 3 to 4-mm thick are produced and analyzed precisely in the way previously described. One must keep in mind that the radiograph of the mastectomy specimen and the radiograph of the slices will be taken in two different orthogonal planes. The macroscopic image of the slices needs to be correlated with both the mediolateral and craniocaudal mammographic projection images.

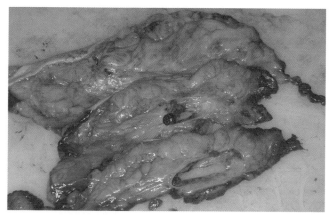

Fig. 8.**15**

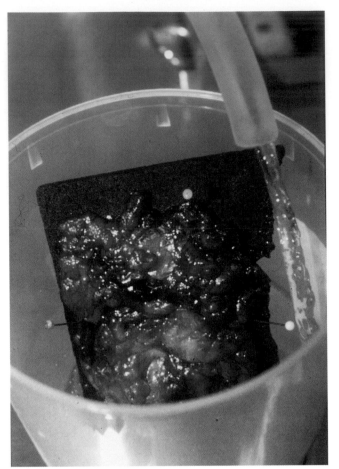

Fig. 8.**16**

Tissue Processing

The selected tissue slices are stretched on a cork plate and pinned, with the surface to be cut facing down. The slices are immersed in dishes containing standard formalin solution for tissue fixation (Fig. 8.**16**). By fixing the tissue when it is stretched, a fairly flat surface can be achieved. The slices are then fixed for 24 hours. Thorough fixation of the slices is essential in this technique; suboptimal fixation causes difficulties on sectioning. Microwave treatment can considerably diminish the time necessary for optimal fixation, but routines must be developed in every laboratory that uses this sensible and particularly useful technique. After fixation, the slices are removed from the cork plate and placed into special-sized container in an automatic tissue processor. Before processing, slices that are already fixed can be trimmed to get the ideal thickness of 3 to 4 mm throughout the whole slice.

Sectioning of the large blocks (Figs. 8.**17** and 8.**19**) is carried out using a special microtome. The most important factor in obtaining large histologic sections of proper quality is the skillful and experienced technician.

Staining is carried out using modified holders, which are placed in the same automatic stainer used for small blocks. The recipe for hematoxylin and eosin staining is the same as for small blocks.

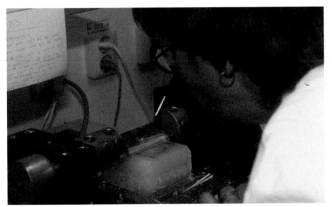

Fig. 8.**17**

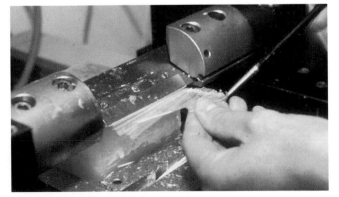

Fig. 8.**18**

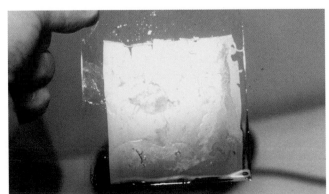

Fig. 8.**19**

Summary of the Steps of Macroscopic Examination

I. Nonmastectomy Specimen

1. Study of the radiograph of the intact surgical specimen
2. Inspection and description of the whole specimen
3. Measurement of the whole specimen
4. Palpation of the specimen
5. Slicing of the specimen into slices 3 to 4-mm thick, parallel with the plane of the mammogram of the intact specimen
6. Placing of the thin slices sequentially on plastic films
7. Macroscopic examination of the cut surfaces of the slices
8. Measurement of the largest tumor dimensions
9. Sampling or aspirating of material for cytologic examinations
10. Marking the suture position with ink
11. Covering the slices with film and marking them with numbers
12. Second specimen radiograph of the slices
13. Comparison of the radiologic and macroscopic abnormalities
14. Selection of the most representative slices
15. Sampling of small blocks for additional methods (in macroscopically detectable lesions larger than 10 mm)

II. Mastectomy Specimen

1–4. As for a nonmastectomy specimen
5.   Slicing of the specimen sagitally
6–15. As for a nonmastectomy specimen

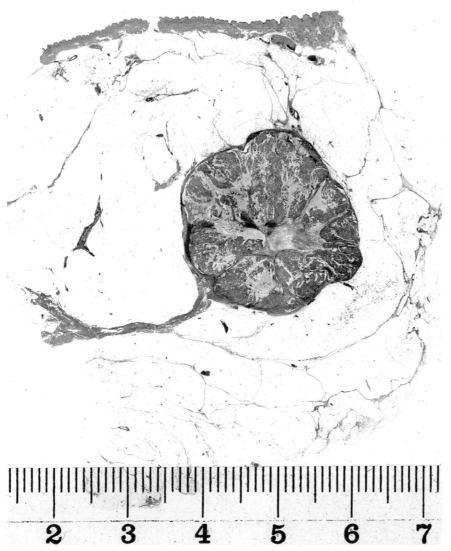

Fig. 8.**20**

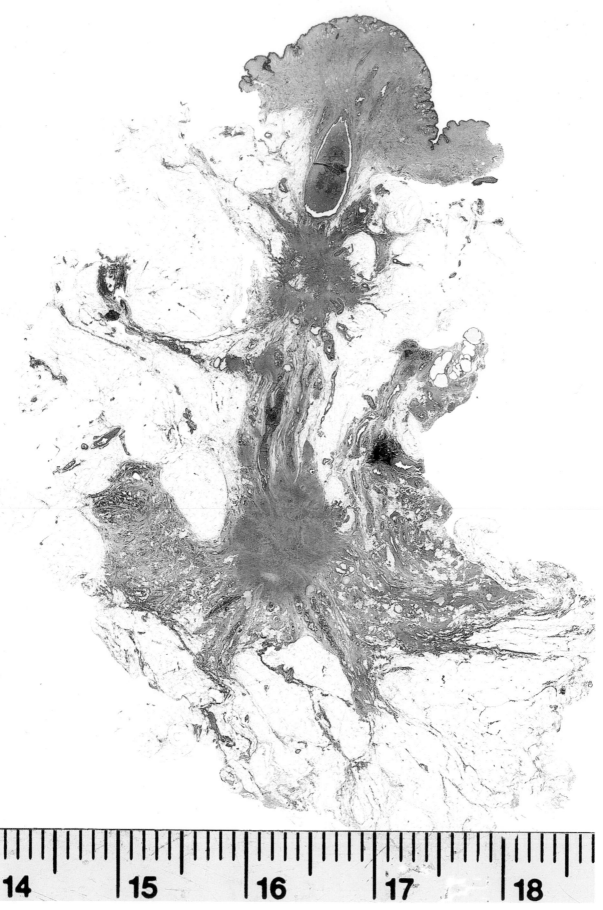

Fig. 8.21

Advantages of the Large-Section Technique

1. Demonstrates the entire lesion in one or several sections, which allows for:
   - ❑ documentation of the tumor size
   - ❑ assessment of the intratumoral heterogeneity
   - ❑ assessment of the effects of diagnostic and/or therapeutic procedures

2. Demonstrates the tumor together with its environment, enabling:
   - ❑ documentation of the multiplicity (multifocality/multicentricity) of the tumor
   - ❑ assessment of the in situ components within and surrounding the tumor
   - ❑ assessment of the relation of the tumor to surrounding benign changes and normal tissue

3. Demonstrates a large area of the resection margins for direct:
   - ❑ assessment of the completeness (radicality) of the excision
   - ❑ measurement of the distance of the tumor from the margin
   - ❑ demonstration of malignant or premalignant changes on the margin

4. Allows a direct correlation of the histologic findings with the mammographically suspicious findings

Conclusions

Large histologic sections demonstrate properly the size, extent, and distribution of breast carcinoma, all in the same histologic section. This technique is a prerequisite for successful clinical, mammographic, and histologic correlation.

References

1   Jackson PA, et al. A comparison of large block macrosectioning and conventional techniques in breast pathology. *Virchows Arch.* 1994;425:243–248.
2   Foschini MP, Tot T, Eusebi V. Large sections (macrosections) from breast tissue. In: Silverstein M, ed. *Ductal carcinoma in situ.* In press.

Chapter 9

Assessment of the Most Important Prognostic Factors

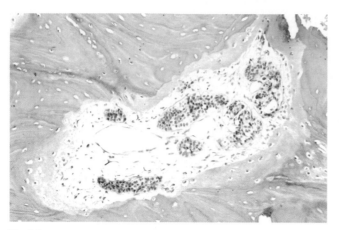

Fig. 9.**1**

Histologic typing of breast carcinomas is an important prognostic factor. However, most invasive tumors belong to the category of ductal, not otherwise specified (NOS) carcinomas. This large and prognostically heterogeneous tumor group needs to be stratified using *morphologic-prognostic factors*. Assessment of these factors is recommended not only for cases of ductal NOS carcinomas but also for all cases of breast carcinomas.

The presence of *distant metastasis* is the most powerful prognostic factor (Fig. 9.**1**).

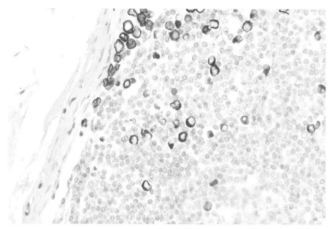

Fig. 9.**2**

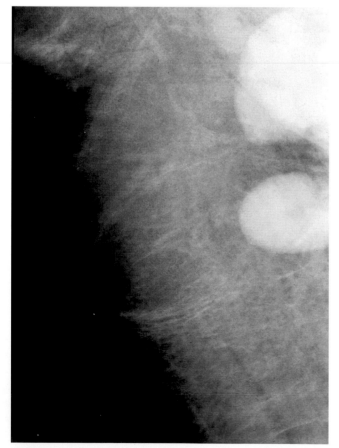

Fig. 9.**3**

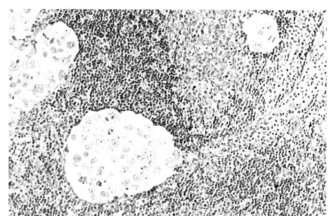

Fig. 9.**4**

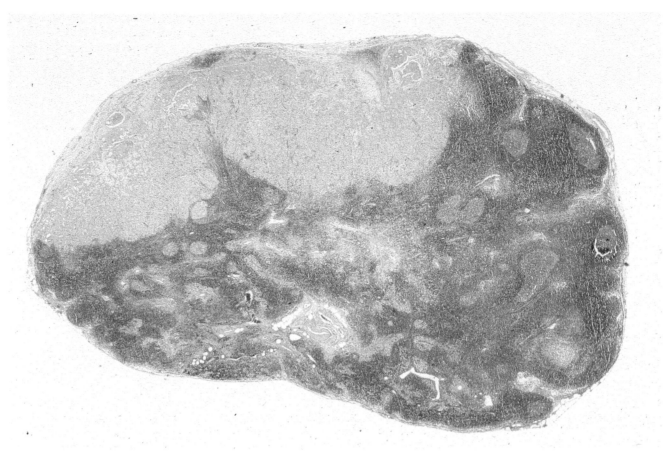

Fig. 9.**5**

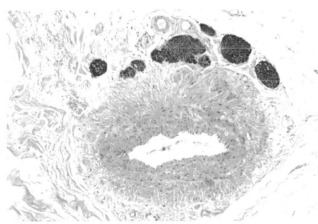

Fig. 9.**6**

The presence of *metastasis in axillary lymph nodes* (Figs. 9.**2** and 9.**5**) is also a powerful prognostic factor and important for therapeutic decision-making. The presence of more than three involved nodes and periglandular infiltration are additional negative prognostic factors. The clinical importance of micrometastases (less than 2 mm) is questioned. The first target of lymphatic spread, the so-called sentinel nodes, may be used as an indicator of the presence of axillary lymph node metastases.

Peritumoral or intratumoral *vascular invasion* (Fig. 9.**6**) usually indicates that metastases are present in the lymph nodes.

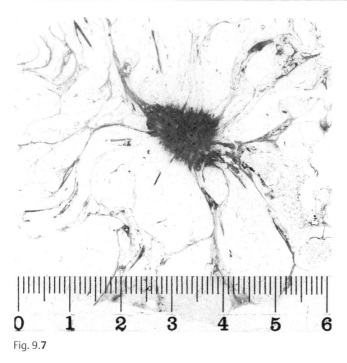

Fig. 9.**7**

The next most powerful prognostic factor is *the size of the tumor*, defined as *the largest diameter of the largest invasive focus.*

Most of the measuring systems accepted by oncologists (e.g., TNM classification) determine the tumor size on macroscopic examination. The macroscopic size of the largest invasive focus correlates very closely with both the mammographic size and the tumor size as measured by ultrasonography. These methods all evaluate the central body of the tumor, which is a parameter representative of tumor cell mass and which correlates with patient survival (Fig. 9.**8**).

A histologic large section taken in the plane of the largest tumor diameter provides medical documentation of the tumor size (Fig. 9.**7**), allowing retrospective and reproducible measurement. Comparison of mammographic, ultrasonographic, and macroscopic tumor size is essential when assessing the histologic size of the tumor. In cases of round or oval tumors (Fig. 9.**10**) the comparison is relatively easy and usually without discrepancies. In cases of stellate tumors, however, the tumor body should be measured histologically without the extensions; otherwise, the histologic size becomes disproportionately larger as compared with the mammographic or ultrasonographic measurements or macroscopic size. The extensions contain a relatively low number of tumor cells, and they do not represent a prognostically important aspect of the tumor.

In cases with more than one clearly formed tumor body (Fig. 9.**9**), the size of the largest tumor is measured separately from the others.

Long-term survival by tumor size

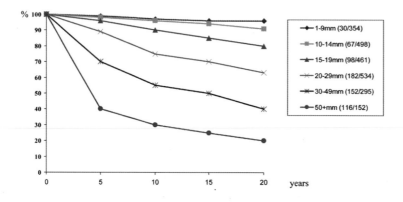

- 1-9mm (30/354)
- 10-14mm (67/498)
- 15-19mm (98/461)
- 20-29mm (182/534)
- 30-49mm (152/295)
- 50+mm (116/152)

Fig. 9.**8** (reproduced from reference no. 4 with permission of the publisher)

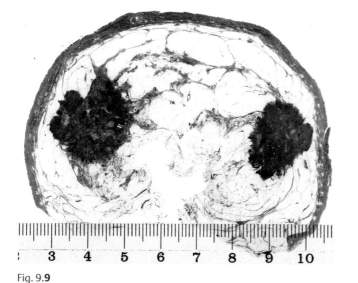

Fig. 9.**9**

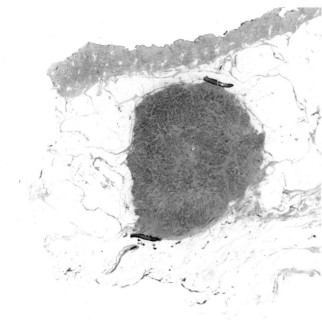

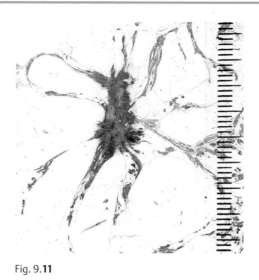

Fig. 9.**11**

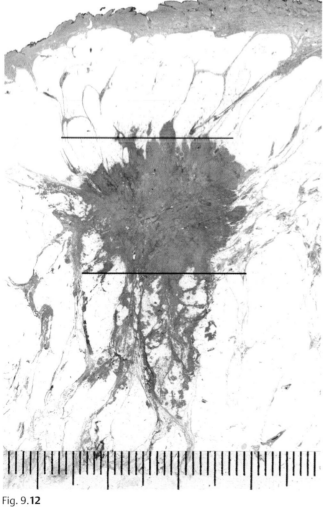

Fig. 9.**10**

The tumors on Figures 9.**10** and 9.**11** are not the same size, although if the extensions are measured and included, both tumors would measure 30 mm. The correct way to assess tumor size histologically is demonstrated in Figure 9.**12**. This can be compared with the erroneous assessment shown in Figure 9.**13**.

Fig. 9.**12**

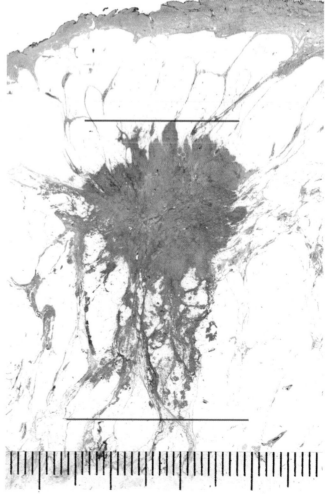

Fig. 9.**13**

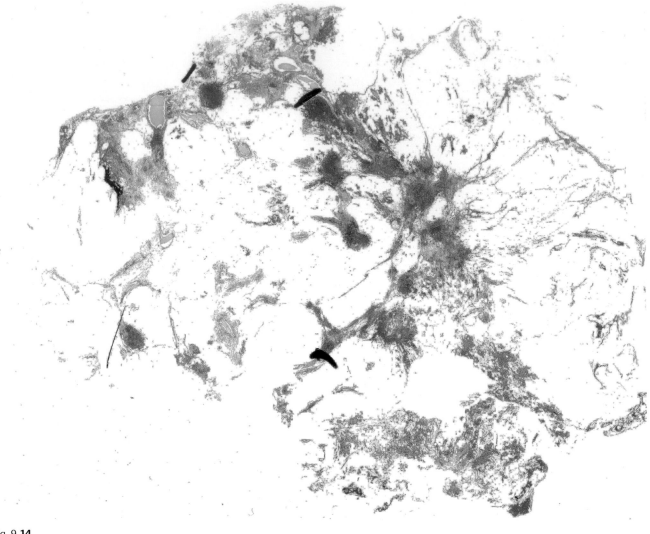

Fig. 9.**14**

Measurement of the area including all the invasive and in situ tumor foci provides another parameter, the *extent of the tumor*. It is measured in two dimensions as distances between the most distant tumor cells, irrespective of whether the cells are in an in situ portion of the tumor, in a body of an invasive tumor or in its extension, or within a lumen of a lymph vessel. The category of *breast carcinoma of limited extent* has been defined as a tumor having no invasive carcinoma, in situ carcinoma, or lymphatic emboli farther than 1 cm from the edge of the dominant mass. This category of breast carcinomas is an appropriate candidate for breast-conserving surgery.

On the other hand, in cases of *extensive breast carcinomas* (Fig. 9.**14**) with a greater distance between invasive tumor foci, a seemingly clear margin free of tumor may be created between two invasive or in situ foci. This may represent a risk for insufficient surgical intervention and local tumor recurrence.

Routine use of the technique of large histologic sections (see Chapter 8) is essential for assessing the extent of breast diseases.

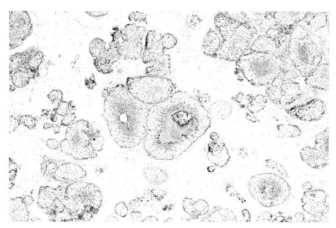

Fig. 9.**15**

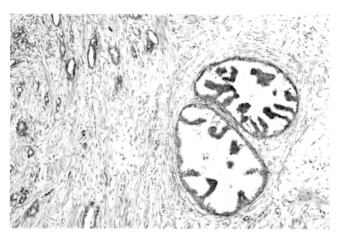

Fig. 9.**16**

The extent of the tumor is not only an important predictor of local recurrence, but is also related to patients' survival. In tumors smaller than 10 mm, the usual prognostic factors, for example tumor grade, are insufficient to stratify the patients into groups with different survivals. The *grade,* and especially the *extent of the associated ductal carcinoma in situ (DCIS),* are newly recognized powerful prognostic factors for these cases (Figs. 9.**15** and 9.**16** illustrate different grades of DCIS associated with invasive cancer). Small invasive tumors associated with extensive grade III DCIS have a significantly less favorable prognosis than the small tumors without extensive DCIS or with extensive DCIS grade I (Fig. 9.**17**). This factor, which can be estimated mammographically as extensive high-grade DCIS, is usually associated with malignant type of microcalcifications ("casting type").

Fig. 9.**17**   (reproduced from reference no. 4 with permission of the publisher)

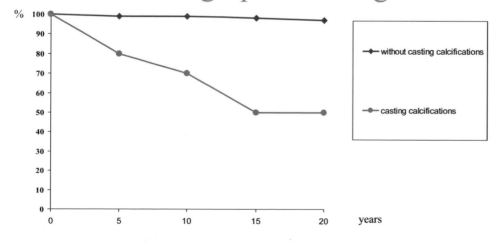

Long-term survival by mammographic findings

- ◆ without casting calcifications
- ● casting calcifications

years

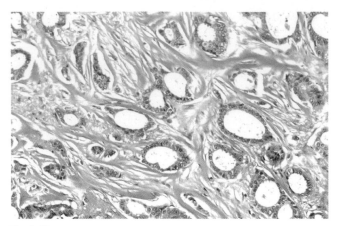

Fig. 9.**18**

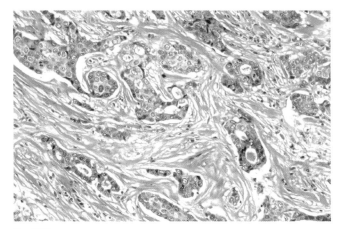

Fig. 9.**19**

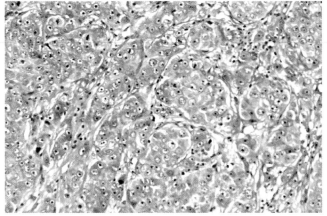

Fig. 9.**20**

The *malignancy grade* of the invasive carcinoma is a powerful prognostic factor in tumors larger than 10 mm (10–15 mm). It can be reproducibly evaluated by using the grading system of Bloom and Richardson, as modified by Elston. This system provides a score (ranging from three to nine points), which sums up the assessment of the tubular structures, the nuclear grade, and the mitotic activity in a representative part of the tumor as follows:

Score 3–5   grade I, well differentiated

Score 6–7   grade II, intermediately differentiated

Score 8–9   grade III, poorly differentiated

Tubular structures (tubule formation) are lumina surrounded by one or more layers of epithelial cells. The assessment is as follows:

– tubules in more than 75% of the tumor   1 (Fig. 9.**18**)

– tubules in 10–75% of the tumor   2 (Fig. 9.**19**)

– tubules in less than 10% of the tumor   3 (Fig. 9.**20**).

The assessment of the *nuclear grade* is similar to the nuclear grading of DCIS. The assessment is as follows:

– small, uniform nuclei   1 (Fig. 9.**22**)

– larger nuclei with visible nucleoli, moderate variability in size and shape   2 (Fig. 9.**24**)

– large, vesicular nuclei with prominent nucleoli and marked variation in size and shape   3 (Fig. 9.**26**)

Mitotic figures are counted per 10 high-power fields at the tumor periphery. Only typical mitotic figures should be counted. The score depends on the field diameter of the microscope used, and the cut-off points have to be adjusted according to the optical parameters.

In this grading system, the tubular structures are relatively easy to assess. Careful counting of mitotic figures is a necessary part of the assessment. However, the nuclear grade is the least reproducible parameter of the system. The grading can be assisted with computer-guided image analysis, which is demonstrated in Figures 9.21, 9.23, and 9.25. The normal epithelial cell nuclei (dark blue column left) are compared with nuclei assessed as nuclear grade I (Fig. 9.21), II (Fig. 9.23), or III (Fig. 9.25). The higher nuclear grade contains larger and more polymorphous nuclei.

A simple way to reach higher intraobserver and interobserver agreement is to compare the diameter of the tumor cell nuclei to a histologic detail of constant diameter (e.g., a red blood cell or a lymphocyte). In cases of nuclear grade I, the tumor nuclei should not have a diameter larger than about two erythrocytes. In grade III, however, tumor cell nuclei with diameters larger than three erythrocytes occur frequently.

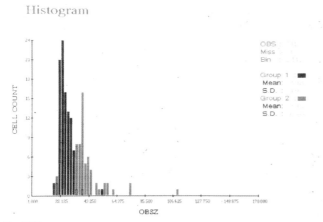

Fig. 9.21

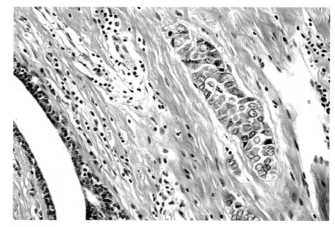

Fig. 9.22

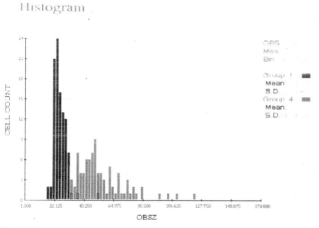

Fig. 9.23

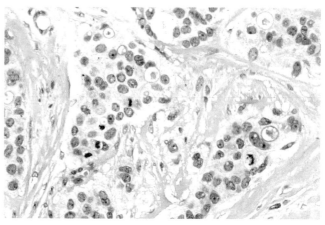

Fig. 9.24

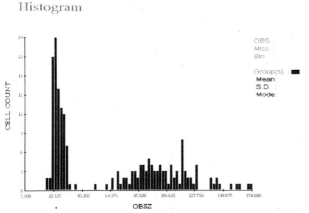

Fig. 9.25

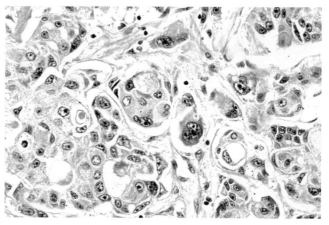

Fig. 9.26

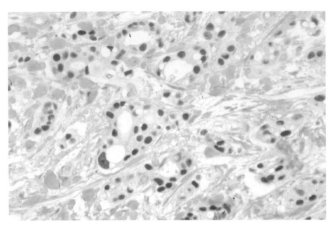

Fig. 9.**27**

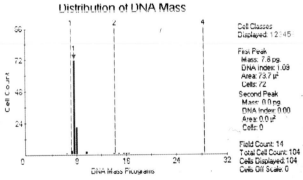

Fig. 9.**28**

Estrogen (and progesterone) receptor status is a prognostic factor as well as a therapeutic one. Expression of the receptors by tumor cell nuclei indicates that the tumor has a high sensitivity to antihormonal therapy.

Hormone receptors are preferably demonstrated and assessed by immunohistochemistry on a histologic section containing tumor tissue and surrounding normal epithelial structures. Automation and external quality control of immunostaining may enhance the reproducibility of the results.

Although most of the tumors are obviously receptor-positive (Fig. 9.**27**), it is necessary to count the ratio of positively stained nuclei to all tumor cell nuclei in some cases. The proposed cut-off point for positivity is 10%.

A negative staining result can be accepted only in the presence of positive controls, preferably the nuclei of the normal tissue in the same section (Fig. 9.**28**).

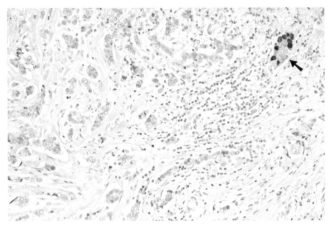

Fig. 9.**29**

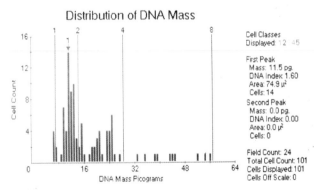

Fig. 9.**30**

Several other prognostic factors are p53, Ki67, DNA analysis (Figs. 9.**29** and 9.**30**), S-phase, c-Erb-B2 (Fig. 9.**31**), tumor angioneogenesis, epidermal growth factor receptor, transforming growth factor-a, Cathepsin D, pS2, bcl-2. None of these newer prognostic factors has been shown and accepted to be as accurate as the combination of the primary prognostic factors.

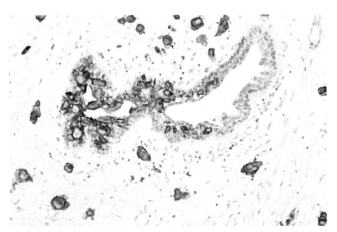

Fig. 9.**31**

Fig. 9.**32** (reproduced from reference no. 4 with permission of the publisher)

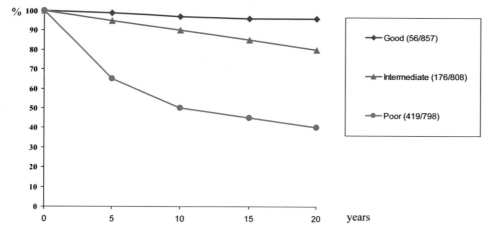

Long-term survival by histological types and grade

Good (56/857)

Intermediate (176/808)

Poor (419/798)

Conclusions

By assessing the main morphologic-prognostic factors (described above), the many variations of breast carcinoma can be stratified into the following three categories, as demonstrated in Figure 9.**32**:

– breast cancer cases with a good prognosis: most in situ carcinomas, tubular carcinomas, mucinous carcinomas, invasive tumors of limited extent, and tumors smaller than 15 mm

– breast cancer cases with a poor prognosis: tumors with metastases, extensive tumors of any size, tumors larger than 20 mm

– breast cancer cases with an intermediate prognosis

Local recurrence is related to the extent and multifocality of the tumor as well as to the radicality of the previous surgical intervention.

Patent survival is related to the stage of the disease: the presence of distant metastases, lymph node status, tumor size, and tumor grade.

References

1 Fitzgibbons PL, et al. Prognostic factors in breast cancer. College of American Pathologists consensus statement 1999. *Arch Pathol Lab Med.* 2000;124:966–978.

2 Elston CW, Ellis JO. Pathological prognostic factors in breast cancer: experience from a long study with long term follow up. *Histopathology.* 1991;19:403–410.

3 Tabár L, et al. A novel method for prediction of long-term outcome of women with T1a, T1b and 10–14-mm invasive breast cancers: a prospective study. *Lancet.* 2000;355(9202):429–433.

4 Tabár L, et al. The Swedish Two-County Trial twenty years later. Updated mortality results and new insights from long-term follow-up. *Radiol Clin North Am.* 2000;38(4):625–651.

5 Faverly DRG, Hendriks JHCL, Holland R. Breast carcinomas of limited extent. Frequency, radiologic-pathologic characteristic, and surgical margin requirements. *Cancer.* 2001;91:647–659.

Chapter 10

Case Reports

Case 1. The Importance of Intratumoral Heterogeneity

This patient was an 80-year-old woman with a large, palpable, rapidly growing lump that filled her right breast (Fig. 10.1.1).

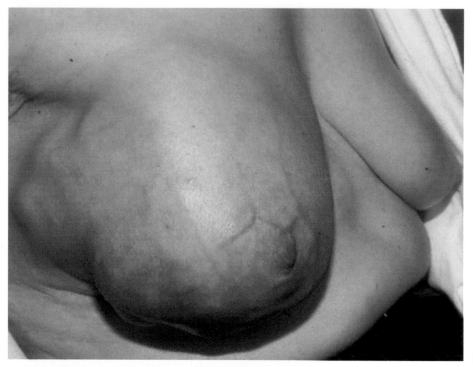

Fig. 10.1.1

Mammography and ultrasonography demonstrated a 7 cm large malignant tumor (Figs. 10.1.2 and 10.1.3).

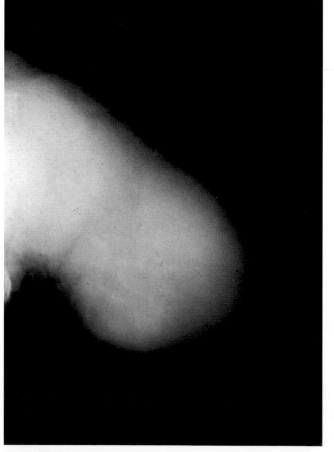

Fig. 10.1.2

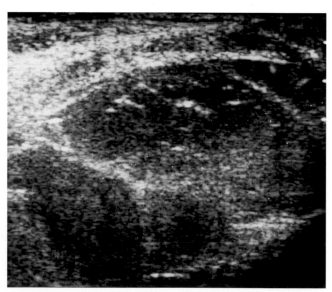

Fig. 10.1.3

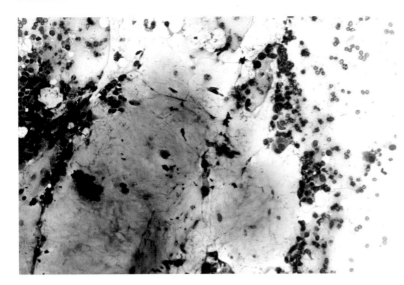

Fig. 10.**1.4**

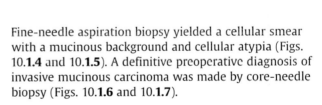

Fig. 10.**1.5**

Fine-needle aspiration biopsy yielded a cellular smear with a mucinous background and cellular atypia (Figs. 10.**1.4** and 10.**1.5**). A definitive preoperative diagnosis of invasive mucinous carcinoma was made by core-needle biopsy (Figs. 10.**1.6** and 10.**1.7**).

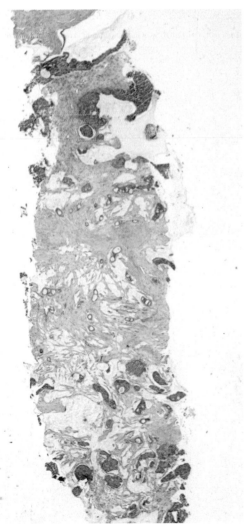

Fig. 10.**1.6**

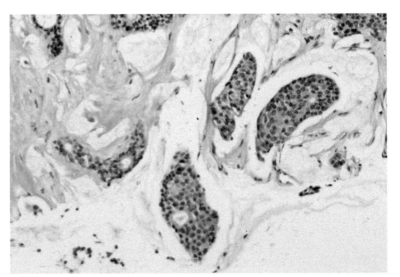

Fig. 10.**1.7**

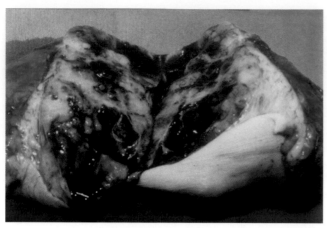

Fig. 10.**1.8**

Mastectomy was performed and a large tumor with a partly hemorrhagic cut surface was macroscopically evident (Fig. 10.**1.8**). On the histologic large section, nearly the entire cut surface could be seen (Fig. 10.**1.9**). Almost 90% of the tumor exhibited the typical picture of mucinous carcinoma with groups of well-differentiated tumor cells floating in a large amount of mucin (Fig. 10.**1.10**). However, an area (about 20 x 10 mm) of more solid tumor tissue was also evident.

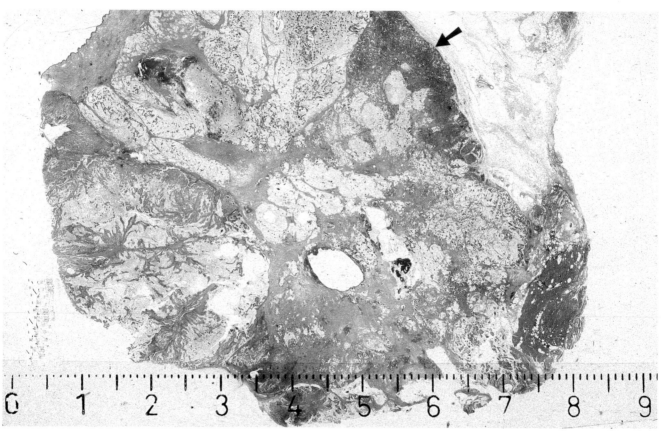

Fig. 10.**1.9**

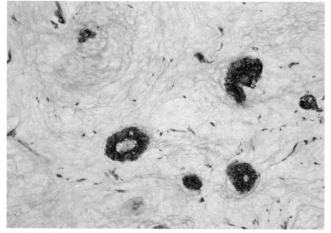

Fig. 10.**1.10**

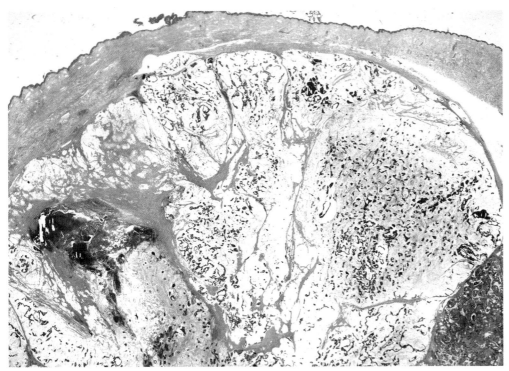

Fig. 10.**1.11**

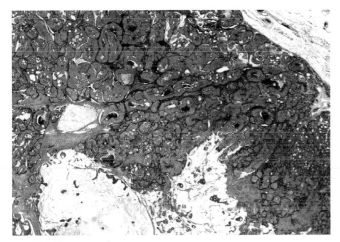

Fig. 10.**1.12**

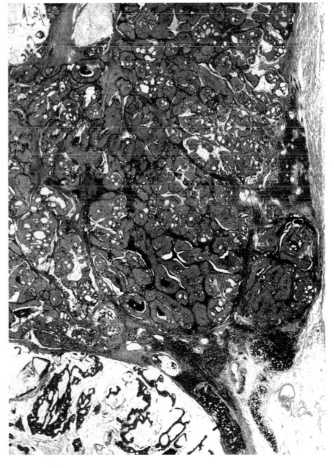

The solid part of the tumor was clearly different from the mucinous component. The cells were poorly differentiated and formed solid nests with central necrosis (Figs. 10.**1.11** and 10.**1.13**). The pattern corresponds to a poorly differentiated, grade III ductal carcinoma.

Fig. 10.**1.13**

The grade III component of the tumor infiltrated the pectoralis muscle (Fig. 10.**1.14**). Lymph vessel invasion was verified (Fig. 10.**1.15**), and the cancer had metastasized to one of the nine examined lymph nodes (Fig. 10.**1.16**).

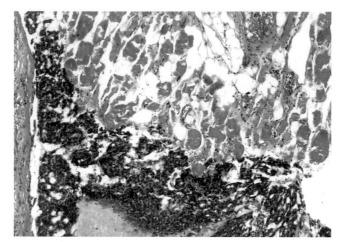

Fig. 10.**1.14**

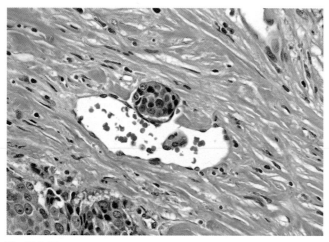

Fig. 10.**1.15**

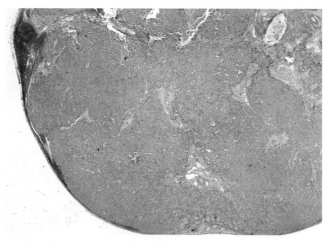

Fig. 10.**1.16**

Conclusions

Although the tumor fulfilled the criteria for mucinous carcinoma (grade I tumor with a mucinous pattern in 90% of the histologic picture), it did not follow the natural history typical of mucinous carcinomas. The outcome will be determined by the minor grade III component.

A thorough postoperative work-up should include a search for evidence of intratumoral heterogeneity.

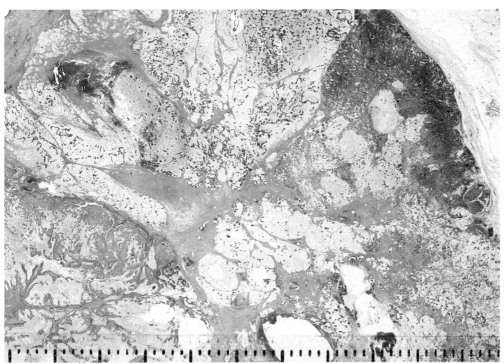

Fig. 10.**1.17**

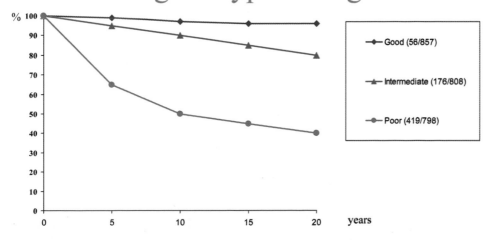

Fig. 10.**1.18**   (the same as 9.32)

Case 2. Breast Carcinoma of Limited Extent (Unifocal Tumor)

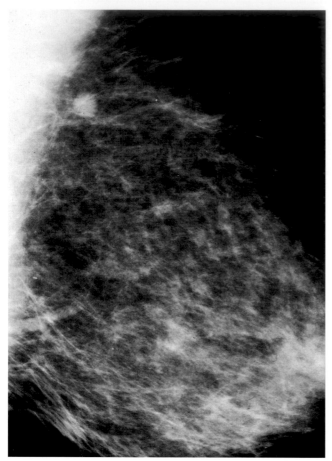

A malignant breast lesion was detected by mammographic screening in a 56-year-old asymptomatic woman (Fig. 10.**2.1**). Ultrasound-guided fine-needle aspiration biopsy (FNAB) yielded a cellular smear without myoepithelial cells and with a large number of noncohesive epithelial cell groups (Fig. 10.**2.2**). The epithelial cells exhibited moderate atypia (Fig. 10.**2.3**). The preoperative cytologic diagnosis was malignant breast tumor.

The large histologic section (Fig. 10.**2.4**) demonstrated that the 7-mm tumor was unifocal invasive ductal carcinoma with an in situ component.

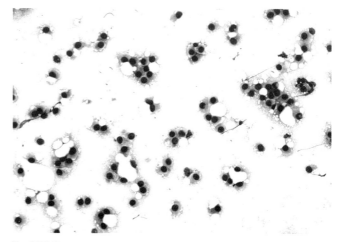

Fig. 10.**2.1**

Fig. 10.**2.2**

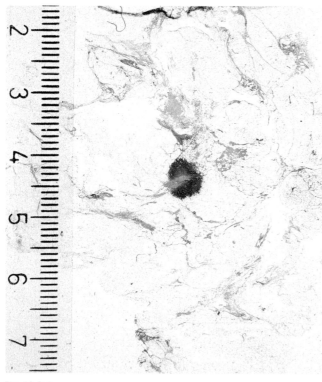

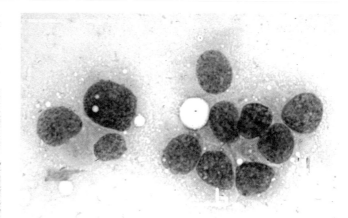

Fig. 10.**2.3**

Fig. 10.**2.4**

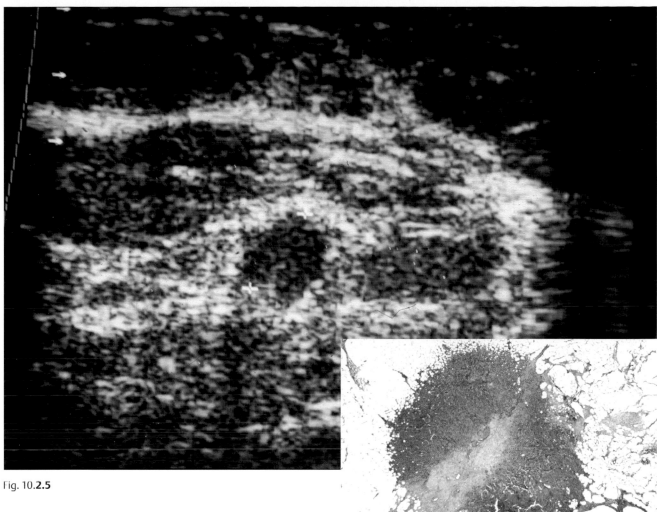

Fig. 10.**2.5**

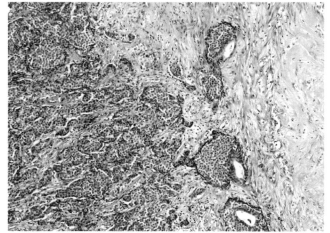

Fig. 10.**2.6**

The tumor clearly showed a central fibrotic area resembling a needling artifact; however, the lesion was present on ultrasound before the aspiration was performed (Figs. 10.**2.5** and 10.**2.6**). The tumor was intermediately differentiated (Fig. 10.**2.7**), and the tumor cells were estrogen-receptor positive (Fig. 10.**2.8**).

The patient has been followed for 4 years and the tumor has not recurred.

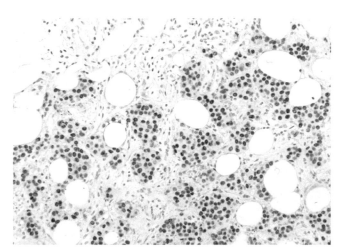

Fig. 10.**2.8**

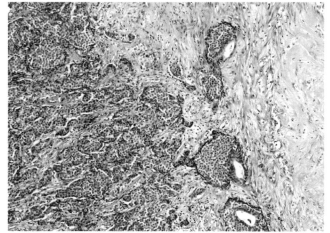

Fig. 10.**2.7**

Conclusions

It is important to determine the size, distribution, and extent of the breast carcinoma because small, unifocal invasive carcinomas without an extensive in situ component have an excellent prognosis.

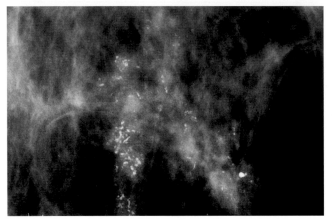

Fig. 10.**3.1**

Case 3. Extensive Breast Carcinoma

A 55-year-old woman presented with a mammographically detected nonpalpable tumor. In addition to the well-formed, small tumor mass, the mammogram showed a large area of microcalcifications of the casting type (Figs. 10.**3.1** and 10.**3.2**). Core biopsy was performed and contained only structures of ductal carcinoma in situ (DCIS) (Figs. 10.**3.3** and 10.**3.4**).

The correlation of mammographic and histologic findings using the large-section technique revealed a large area of DCIS grade III. In this area, a 9-mm grade III invasive ductal carcinoma was also seen (Figs. 10.**3.5** and 10.**3.6**).

The diagnosis of extensive ductal carcinoma grade III was established: the tumor size was 9 mm and the extent 50 x 30 mm.

Fig. 10.**3.2**

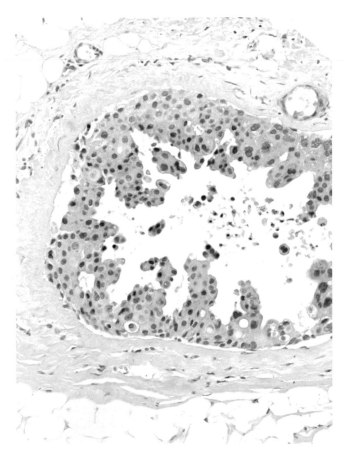

Fig. 10.**3.4**

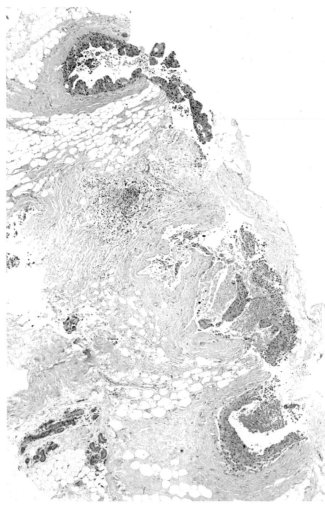

Fig. 10.**3.3**

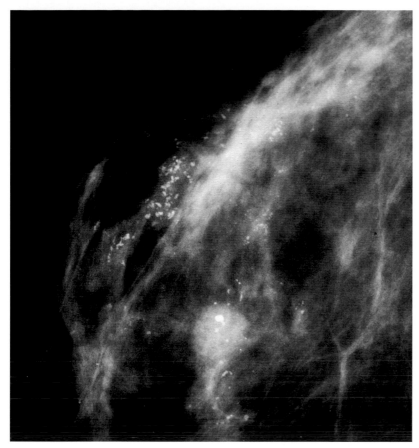

Fig. 10.**3.5**

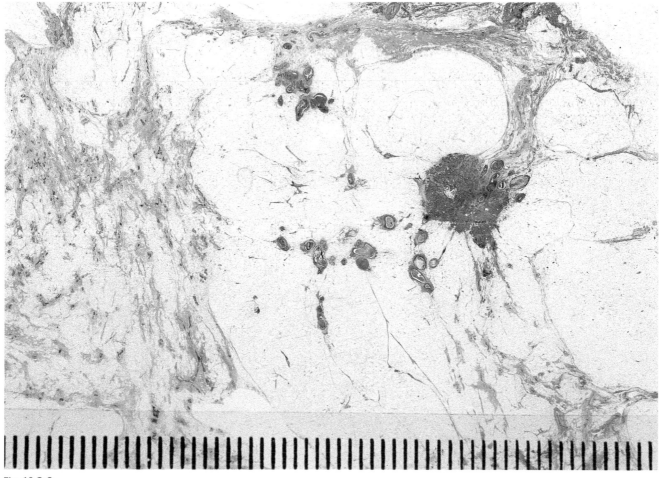

Fig. 10.**3.6**

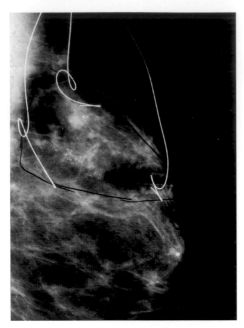

Fig. 10.**3.7**

Further details of the invasive and in situ component of the tumor are shown in Figures 10.**3.7**–10.**3.12**. The periductal inflammation and fibrosis, which are possible indirect signs of duct neogenesis, can be seen.

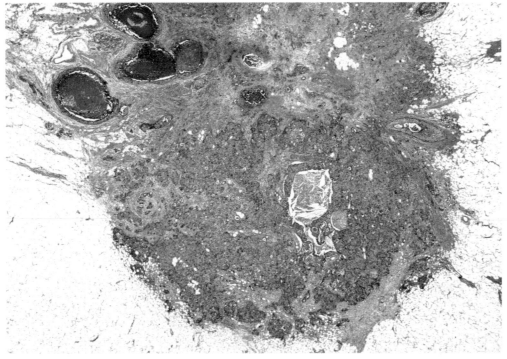

Fig. 10.**3.8**

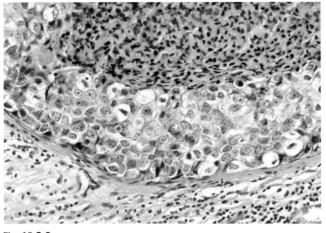

Fig. 10.**3.9**

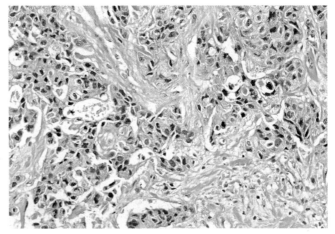

Fig. 10.**3.10**

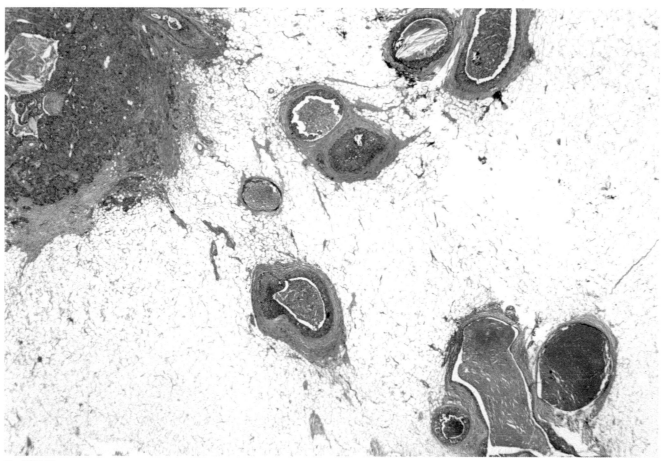

Fig. 10.**3.11**

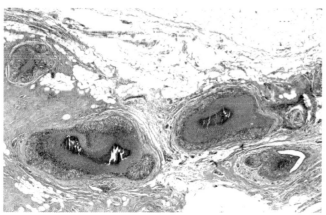

Fig. 10.**3.12**

As shown in Figure 10.**3.13**, the patient had lymph node metastases in three of the 10 examined nodes. There have been no signs of recurrence during the follow-up period of 2 years.

Conclusions

Careful assessment of the extent of the disease is an important part of the postoperative work-up because patients with extensive breast carcinomas, especially associated with grade III DCIS, have worse prognosis than patients with breast carcinomas of the same size and grade, but of limited extent (Fig. 10.**2.14**).

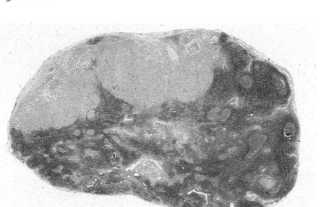

Fig. 10.**3.13**

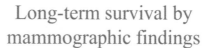

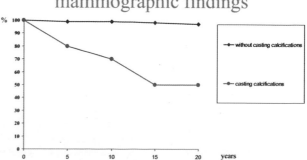

Fig. 10.**3.14**   (the same as 9.17)

Case 4. Extensive Invasive Lobular Carcinoma

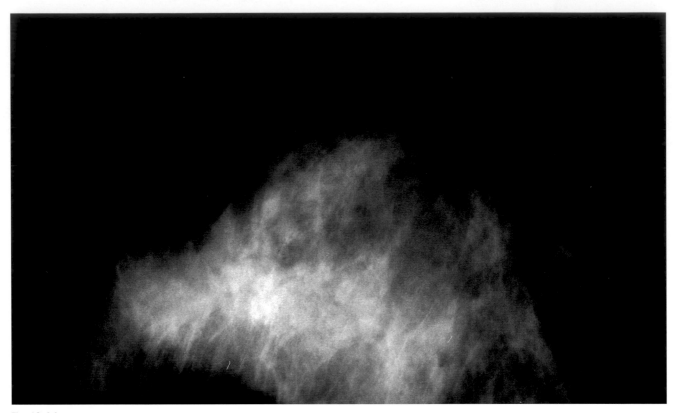

Fig. 10.**4.1**

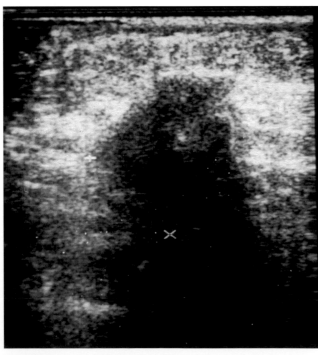

Fig. 10.**4.2**

This patient presented clinically with a large, diffuse, palpable lesion. Both the mammogram and ultrasound examination demonstrated a large malignant tumor (Figs. 10.**4.1** and 10.**4.2**). Fine-needle aspiration, however, yielded a smear with only a few groups of small, regular cells (Fig. 10.**4.3**).

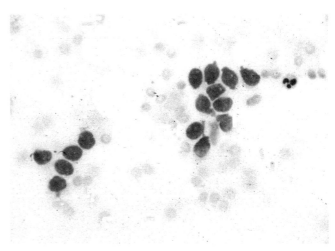

Fig. 10.**4.3**

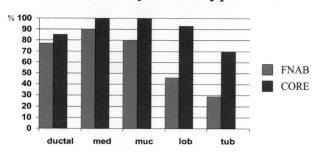

Fig. 10.**4.4** (the same as 7.**27**)

Core biopsy allowed the definitive preoperative diagnosis of invasive lobular carcinoma to be established (Figs. 10.**4.5**–10.**4.7**). As discussed in Chapter 7, one of the advantages of core biopsy compared with FNAB is a higher accuracy in making the preoperative diagnosis of invasive lobular carcinoma (Fig. 10.**4.4**).

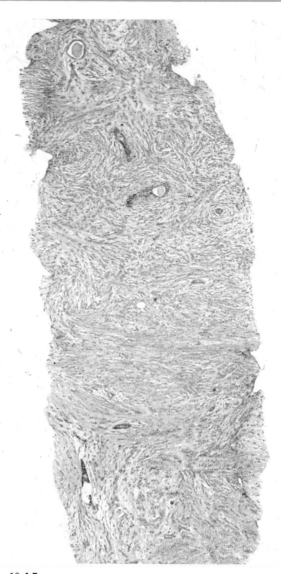

Fig. 10.**4.5**

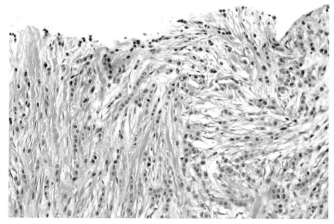

Fig. 10.**4.6**

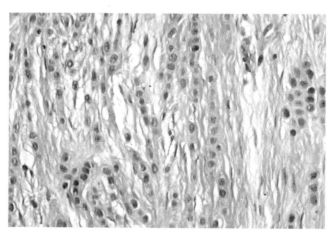

Fig. 10.**4.7**

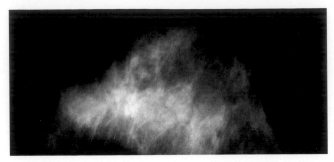

Fig. 10.**4.8**

Large-section histology (Fig. 10.**4.9**) showed an area of at least 50 x 30 mm of invasive lobular carcinoma, mainly of the classic type, with some intratumoral heterogeneity (Figs. 10.**4.10**–10.**4.12**). Four of the examined axillary lymph nodes contained metastases (Fig. 10.**4.13**). The patient died of metastatic breast carcinoma 3 years later.

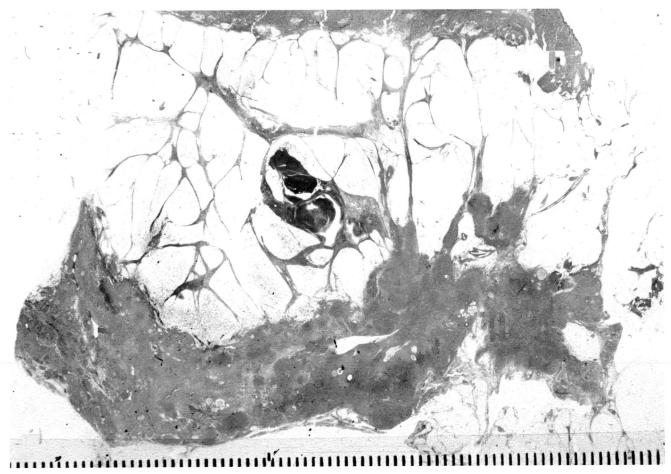

Fig. 10.**4.9**

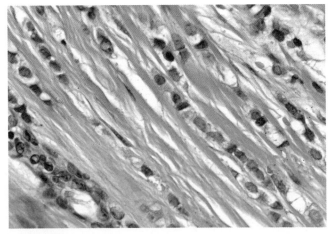

Fig. 10.**4.10**

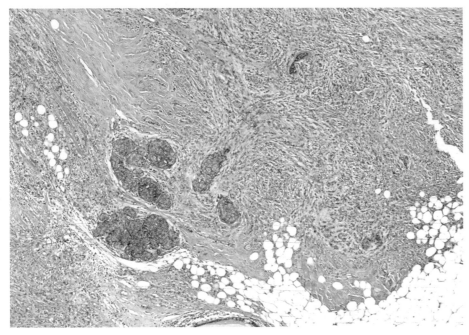

Fig. 10.**4.11**

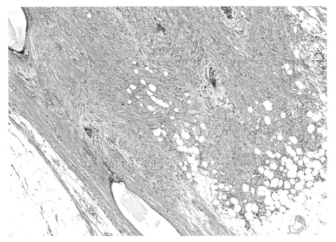

Fig. 10.**4.12**

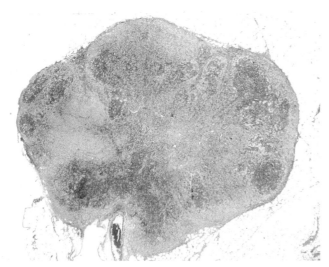

Fig. 10.**4.13**

Conclusions

Invasive lobular carcinoma may exhibit a diffuse growth pattern. These tumors are extensive, aggressive, and have a poor prognosis.

Case 5. Breast Carcinoma of Limited Extent?

A 60-year-old asymptomatic woman presented with a unifocal stellate lesion detected by mammographic screening (Fig. 10.**5.1**), which was well visualized by ultrasonography (Fig. 10.**5.2**). The lesion was seen on the mammogram as a white star with a well-formed tumor body.

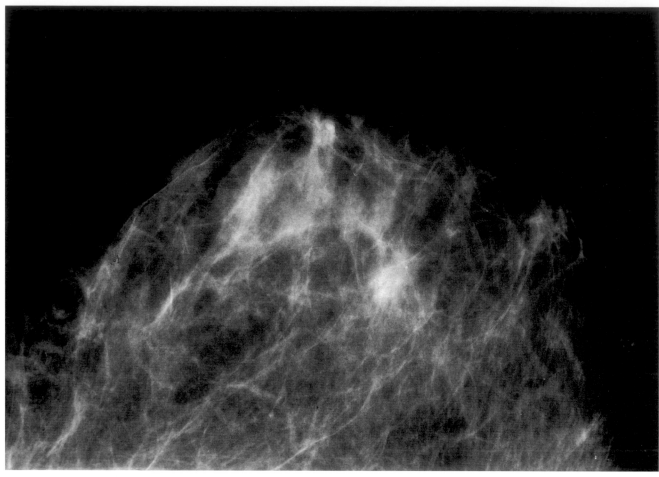

Fig. 10.**5.1**

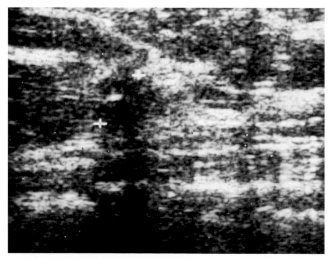

Fig. 10.**5.2**

Ultrasound-guided fine-needle aspiration was performed and yielded a moderately cellular smear with some cell groups with atypia (Fig. 10.**5.4**). The cytological picture was categorized as IV, suspicious for malignancy.

Diagnostic accuracy of FNAB in 240 breast cancers

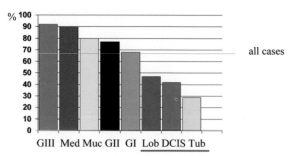

Fig. 10.**5.3** (the same as 7.**21**)

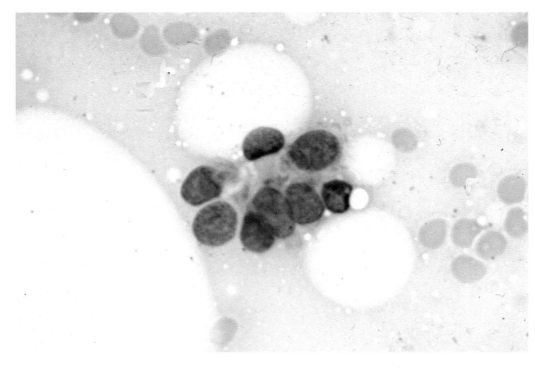

Fig. 10.**5.4**

As mentioned in Chapter 7, FNAB is not an effective way of diagnosing tubular carcinoma (Fig. 10.**5.3**).

Preoperative core biopsy was indicated to confirm the malignant nature of the lesion. The core was representative and included tumor structures in an area of in situ carcinoma and normal structures (Fig. 10.**5.5**). To confirm the invasive character of the tubular structures, immunohistochemical staining on smooth muscle actin was performed (Fig. 10.**5.6**).

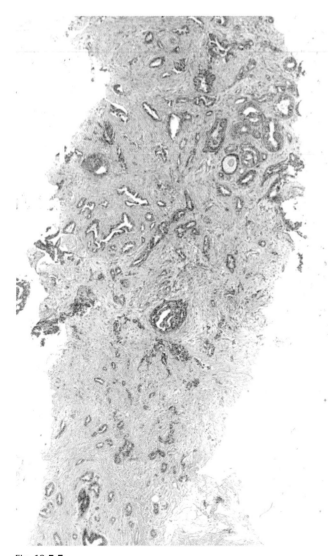

Fig. 10.**5.5**

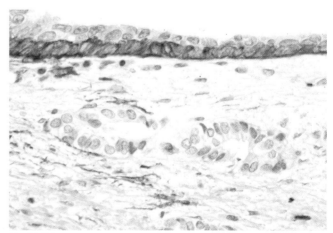

Fig. 10.**5.6**

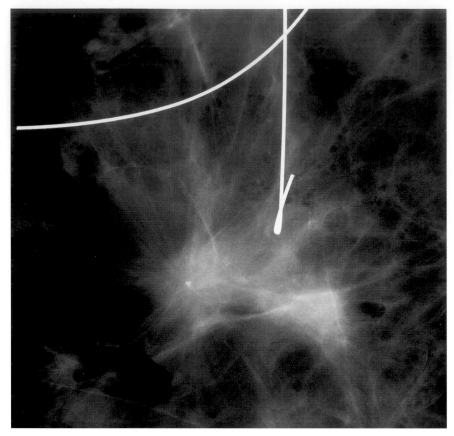

Fig. 10.**5.7**

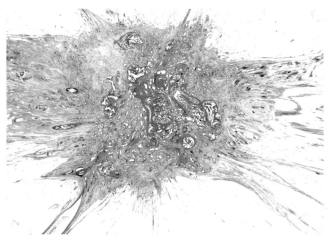

Fig. 10.**5.8**

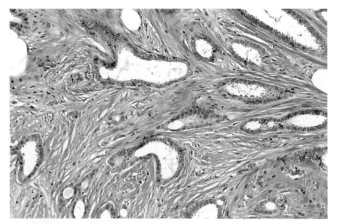

Fig. 10.**5.9**

By correlating the mammographic findings with the large histologic section, the solitary 8-mm stellate lesion could be easily recognized corresponding to invasive tubular carcinoma (Figs. 10.**5.7**–10.**5.10**) and containing structures of DCIS grade I within the tumor.

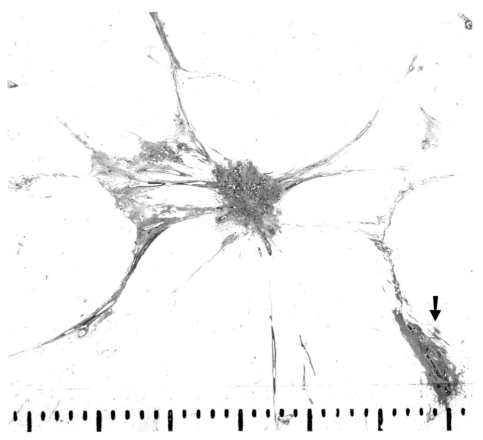

Fig. 10.**5.10**

As a more sensitive method than radiology, histology revealed a 3-mm focus fulfilling the criteria of DCIS grade I (Fig. 10.**5.10** and the corresponding magnification in Fig. 10.**5.11**) at a distance of 30 mm from the dominant tumor mass and very near the circumferential resection margin.

Another completing surgical excision was done but the excised tissue did not contain tumor structures. There have been no signs of recurrence during the 3-year follow-up period.

Conclusions

This case may be diagnosed as breast carcinoma of limited extent, although the proposed criteria (no tumor beyond 1 cm from the edge of the dominant mass) are not fulfilled.

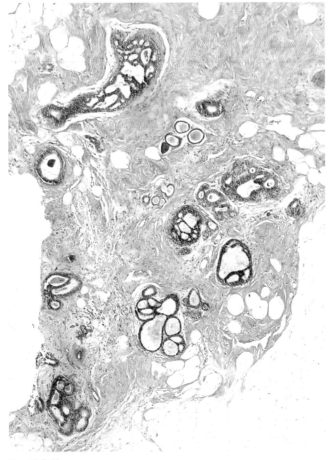

Fig. 10.**5.11**

Case 6. Tumor-Forming DCIS

This 67-year-old woman noted a breast mass. The radiologic examination revealed a stellate tumor mass without signs of multifocality (Fig. 10.**6.1**). She also had palpable lymph nodes in her axilla.

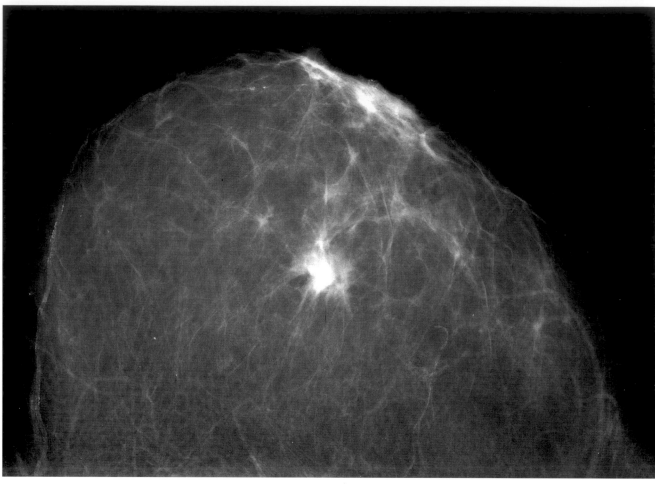

Fig. 10.**6.1**

FNAB yielded a cellular smear with moderate atypia and with a minimal number of myoepithelial cells, categorized as V, malignant (Figs. 10.**6.2** and 10.**6.3**).

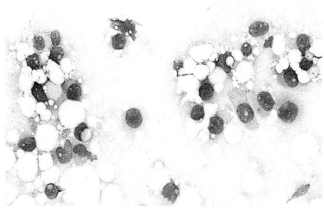

Fig. 10.**6.2**

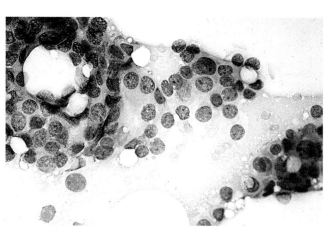

Fig. 10.**6.3**

Segmentectomy and axillary lymph node evacuation were performed. The large histologic section (Fig. 10.**6.4**) demonstrated the solitary 10-mm lesion. At higher magnification (Fig. 10.**6.5**), epithelial displacement as a consequence of a needling procedure was well seen.

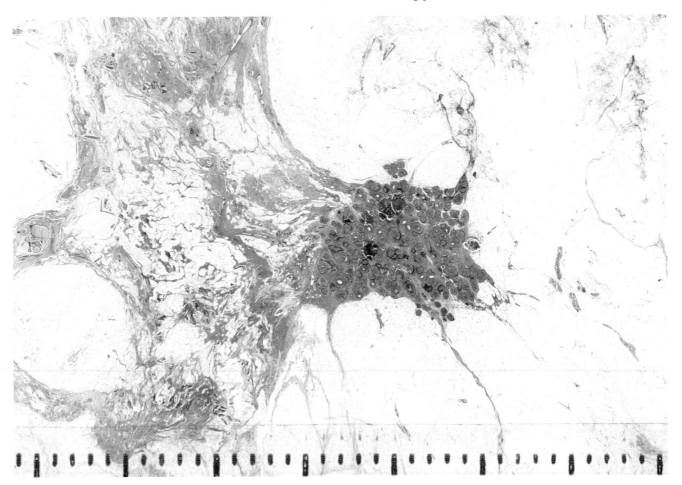

Fig. 10.**6.4**

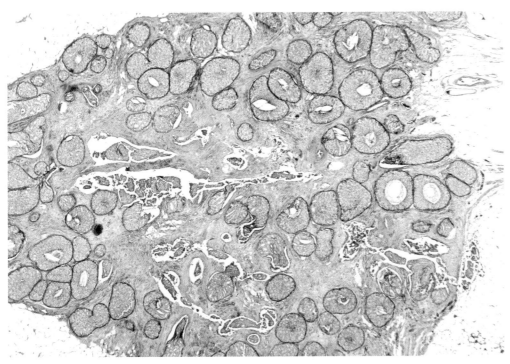

Fig. 10.**6.5**

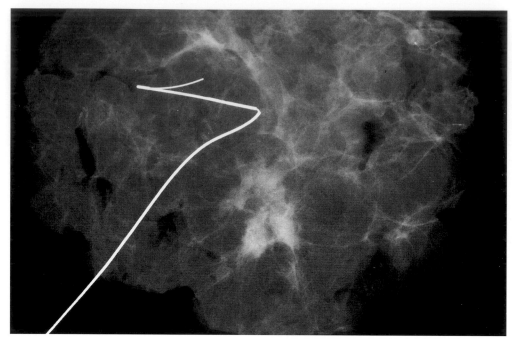

Fig. 10.**6.6**

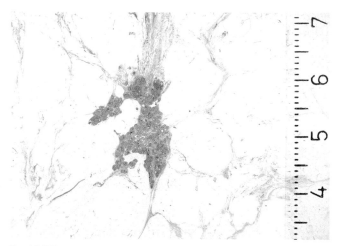

Fig. 10.**6.7**

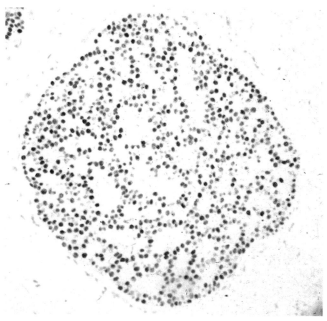

Fig. 10.**6.8**

In another slice of the tumor, the large section revealed that the tumor varied in size and shape (Fig. 10.**6.7**, as compared with Fig. 10.**6.4**). Pseudoinvasion, a consequence of the needling procedure, was also evident. However, the tumor structures had the form of dilated acini and no invasion into the stroma could be demonstrated (Fig. 10.**6.8**). The basement membrane was also seen around the structures (Figs. 10.**6.9** and 10.**6.10**). The lesion was diagnosed as ductal carcinoma in situ, grade I, tumor-forming.

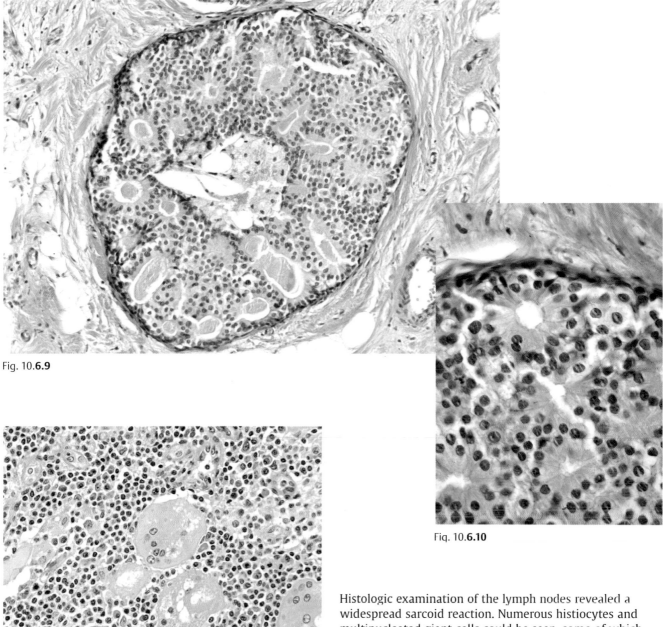

Fig. 10.**6.9**

Fig. 10.**6.10**

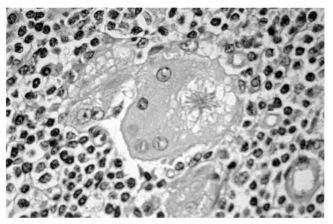

Fig. 10.**6.11**

Histologic examination of the lymph nodes revealed a widespread sarcoid reaction. Numerous histiocytes and multinucleated giant cells could be seen, some of which contained asteroid bodies (Figs. 10.**6.11** and 10.**6.12**).

Conclusions

The rare tumor-forming subtype of DCIS often causes differential diagnostic difficulties. A sarcoid reaction, sometimes seen in lymph nodes draining tumors, may lead to a false clinical impression of the presence of lymph node metastasis.

Fig. 10.**6.12**

Index